# Acupressure for Muscular Dystrophy Made Easy

## An Illustrated Self Treatment Guide

Dr. Krishna N. Sharma

Disclaimer:

Information provided this book is meant to complement and not replace any advice or information from a health professional. The reader is encouraged to use good judgment when applying the information contained and to seek advice from a qualified professional if, and as, needed. The author reserves the right not to be responsible for the topicality, correctness, completeness or quality of the information provided. Liability claims regarding damage caused by the use of any information provided, including any kind of information which is incomplete or incorrect, will therefore be rejected.

Copyright Notice:

Published by the Amazon Group, USA

Copyright © 2013 Dr. Krishna N. Sharma

All rights reserved.

ISBN: 1482099608
ISBN-13: 978-1482099607

# DEDICATION

To my Parents
*Dr. L. Sharma*
*Smt. Chintamani Sharma*

# CONTENTS

# ACKNOWLEDGMENTS

I wish to express my sincere gratitude to my beloved parents and family for their support, strength, love, help and for everything.

I would like to thank all my Muscular Dystrophy Patients who put faith on me and blessed me the opportunity to join the fight against Muscular Dystrophy with them.

Last but not least I wish to avail myself of this opportunity, express a sense of gratitude and love to my friends for their love, encouragement and critical reviews.

# PREFACE

It is my immense pleasure to present my twenty fifth book on Acupressure. This book is a small effort to help the Muscular Dystrophy patients make their life easier. The journey of this book started when I was looking for acupressure books exclusively written to treat the Muscular Dystrophy patients. I searched on various online bookstores, but could not find any appropriate book. It motivated me to write a book which may help the patients, their families and health professionals etc treat the patients. Since I have tried to keep the medical terms away as much as possible and there are lots and lots of illustrations, I hope you'll find it easy to administer.

I hope that this book will help convey to the readers some of the fascination that this subject matter holds for me.

Mumbai, India                    Dr. Krishna N. Sharma
Email:   dr.krisharma@gmail.com
Web: http://www.krishna.info.ms

DR. KRISHNA N. SHARMA

# 1 WHAT IS MUSCULAR DYSTROPHY

Muscular dystrophy (MD) is actually a group of muscle diseases which weakens the muscles and affects the movement.

These are characterized by defects in muscle proteins, progressive muscle weakness (skeletal muscles), and the death of muscle cells and tissue.

**Types:**

These are mainly of the following types-
- Becker muscular dystrophy
- Duchenne muscular dystrophy
- Emery-Dreifuss muscular dystrophy
- Facioscapulohumeral muscular dystrophy
- Limb-girdle muscular dystrophy
- Myotonia congenita
- Myotonic dystrophy

**Symptoms:**

Muscular Dystrophy has a wide range of symptoms. In this book we'll learn how to manage the following symptoms:

a) Neuromuscular Problems-
    i. Paresis / Paralysis
    ii. Limbs' Weakness
    iii. Ataxia
    iv. Incoordination
    v. Difficulty in Speech

b) Psychological and Mental Problems-
    i. Lack of Joy
    ii. Anxiety and Nervousness
    iii. Depression
    iv. Insomnia
    v. Memory And Concentration

c) Digestive Problems-
    i. Constipation

d) Urinary Problems-
    i. Loss of bladder control
    ii. Urinary retention

e) Sexual Problems-
    i. Loss of libido

f) Visual Problems and Nystagmus-

# 2 WHAT IS ACUPRESSURE

Acupressure is an ancient Chinese alternative medicine technique. It is derived from acupuncture. It is based on the Traditional Chinese medicine's (TCM) acupuncture theory developed 5,000 years ago. As the name reflects, it is a technique in which the ailments are treated by applying pressure on specific acu points spread throughout the body. These points are located on imaginary lines called meridians.

These meridians are:
- Lung Meridian
- Large Intestine Meridian
- Stomach Meridian
- Spleen Meridian
- Heart Meridian
- Small Intestine Meridian
- Bladder Meridian
- Kidney Meridian
- Pericardium Meridian

- Triple Warmer Meridian
- Gall Bladder Meridian
- Liver Meridian
- Conception Vessel Meridian
- Governing Vessel Meridian

According to the TCM theory, this technique works by stimulating the meridian system to bring about relief by rebalancing yin, yang and chi (also called "qi").

*Chi* can not be exactly defined but in a way we may call it life force. In Japan it is called *Qi* or *Ki*; In India and Hinduism it is *Prana*; in Arabian countries and Islam it is *Barraka*; in Hebrew it is *Rauch*; Polynesians call it *Mana*.

**Bony Landmarks:**

The bony landmarks are important in term of finding and identifing the acu points.

### *Cranium:*

The main landmarks on the cranium are:

• *Cheekbone and arch (maxillary bone, zygomatic bone, and zygomatic arch):* It runs from the ear to the nose. Firstly start with placing your fingers in front of your ear to palpate the *zygomatic arch* (a part of the temporal bone). Now go tho the downward direction, then you'll feel the *zygomatic bone.* Now curve back up toward your nose to feel the *maxillary bone.*

• *Orbit of the eye (Eye socket)*: To palpate the full orbit, place your fingers on your eyebrows where you can feel the upper border of the orbit. Now run your fingers all along this bony circle.

• *Occipital protuberance:* Put your fingers behind your head and feel the hollow on the junction of the end of skull and the spinal column. Palpate the bony protuberances on either side of the hollow. It is the *Occipital protuberance.*

### Shoulder Blades and Vertebrae:

The main landmarks on the shoulder blade and vertebrae are:

• *Vertebrae:* There are 7 vertebrae in the neck (cervical), 12 vertebrae in the midback where the ribs attached behind (thoracic), and 5 vertebrae in the low back (lumbar).

• *Shoulder Blade (scapula):* The two shoulder blades are placed on each side of your spinal column. These are triangular in shape. We need to palpate 4 main landmarks.

o *Inner border:* It is the edge of the blade closest to the spinal column.
o *Outer border:* It is the outer edge of the shoulder blade.
o *Superior angle:* Follow the inner border upwards and once you reach the sharp point on top of the border.
o *Inferior angle:* This is the lowermost point of the shoulder blade.

### Chest and Shoulder:

The main landmarks on the chest are:

• *Chest bone (sternum):* It is in the bone in the middle of your chest. It has three parts: the upper part which connects with the collarbones (clavicle) is called the *Manubrium*, the middle part is called the *Body*, and the lower little part is called the *zyphoid process.*

• *Collar Bones (clavicals):* These are the horizontal bones connecting the upper part of the chest bone and the point of the shoulder.

• *Point of the shoulder (acromium processes):* This is the point where the collar bones meet the shoulder blades. It can be felt at the top of the shoulder.

### *Arm and Hand:*
The main landmarks on the arm and hand are:

• *Deltoid tuberosity:* It is a bump located on the outside of the upper part of arm bone (where the doctors give injection).

• *Elbow bone (olecranon process):* Bend your elbow and the point of bone you find on the back of elbow is the *olecranon process.*

• *Lateral epicondyle:* Bend your elbow and the point of bony elevation you find on the outer side of the elbow is the *Lateral epicondyle.*
• *Medical epicondyle:* Bend your elbow and the point of bony elevation you find on the inner side of the elbow is the *Medial epicondyle.*

• *Wrist bone (ulnar tuberosity):* You can find it as a bony elevation on the little fingure's side of the back of your wrist.
• *Metacarpals:* These are the five bones that go from the wrist bones to the fingers — just like the metatarsals go from the anklebones to the toes. Feel the areas between the bones where the tendons run. These areas are important for point location.

### *Hip, pelvic, and buttock bones:*
The main landmarks on the Hip, pelvic, and buttock bones are:

• *Hipbone Point (ASIS):* It can be found on either side of the lower stomach.

• *Top of the hipbone (iliac crest):* Move your fingers upward and backward starting from the Hipbone Point (ASIS). The bony border you feel all the way is the *Top of the hipbone (iliac crest).*

• *Pubic bone:* It can be felt between the two Hipbone Point (ASIS).

• *Sacrum:* It is a triangular bone with the vertex downwards at the bottom of your spinal column.

### *Knee bones and joints:*

The main landmarks on the Hip, pelvic, and buttock bones are:

• *Kneecap (patella):* Straighten your leg and place your hand over the upper part of the knee. You can feel a small movable bone. It is the *Kneecap (patella).*

• *Knee bump (tibial tuberosity):* The first bony elevation below the Kneecap (patella) and on the uppermost part of the shinbone is *Knee bump (tibial tuberosity).*

• *Outer side of knee (fibular head):* It can be palpated as a bony elevation on the outer side of the knee joint at almost the same level as the *Knee bump (tibial tuberosity).*

### *Ankle and Foot:*

The main landmarks on the ankle and foot are:

• *The outer anklebone (lateral malleolus):* You can palpate it as a big bony prominance on the outer side of your ankle. It is a part of the fibula bone.

• *Outer leg bone (fibula):* You can palpate it by moving your hand upward from the *outer anklebone (lateral malleolus)* to the knee.

• *Inner anklebone (medial malleolus):* It is situated on the inner side of the ankle just like the *outer anklebone (lateral malleolus)* but on its opposite side.

• *Shinbone (tibia):* It can be palpated on the front of the leg (shin).

**Meridians:**

The meridian is a hypothetical path which is believed to circulate *chi* flows through it.

There are 20 meridians which include 12 *Regular Meridians* and 8 *Extraordinary Meridians*. The 12 Regular Meridians are named by the organs they govern. Six of the Regular Meridians start or stop in the hands, and other six of them start or stop in the feet.

**Cun:**

It is the standard unit of measurement for the body used in acupuncture. It is required to locate the acu points and measure the distance from point.

*One cun:* It is equal to the width of the thumb, in the middle, at the crease.

*One and Half Cun:* It is equal to the combined breadth of two fingers (index and middle).

*Three cun:* It is equal to the combined breadth of the four fingers (except the thumb).

*Twelve cun:* It is equal to the distance from the elbow crease to the wrist crease.

## Pressure Application:

The point should be pressed by finger or some blunt object.

If you get the point correctly, it will feel somewhat different on pressing. You may feel the point sore, tense or aching etc., but it confirms that you are pressing a acu point.

There is no hard and fast rule regarding the amount of pressure, but as per the general guideline, the pressure should be firm enough so that it "hurts good".

There is no hard and fast rule regarding the duration of the pressure applied on the points. But it may range from less than half a second to two minutes.

## Warning:

Do not apply pressure in the following conditions.
- Bleeding
- Bruises
- Contagious Diseases
- Contusions
- Deep emotional trauma
- Fractures
- Infections
- Inflammation (signs of Redness + Swelling + Heat + Dysfunction)
- Prolapsed Intervertebral Disc (PIVD)

- Severe spinal trauma
- Severe swelling (edema)
- Sprains
- Strains
- Surgery
- Varicose Veins

# 3 NEUROMUSCULAR PROBLEMS

Here in this chapter, we'll learn about the acu points to get rid of mainly 7 problems:

a)   Paresis / Paralysis
b)   Limbs' Weakness
c)   Ataxia
d)   Incoordination
e)   Difficulty in Speech

## a) Paresis / Paralysis:

### i) Upper Limb Paresis / Paralysis

**LI4:**
*Location:* It is situated between the 1st and 2nd metacarpal bones on the back side (dorsum) of the hand.

**LI11:**
*Location:* It is situated between LU5 and the lateral epicondyle. You can easily locate it after bending your elbow.

### LI14:

*Location:* It is situated at the inferior border of the deltoid 4 cun above LI13 on the line connecting LI11 and LI15.

### LI15:

*Location:* It is situated on the upper portion of the deltoid muscle, anterior and inferior to the acromion process. It may be found in a depression formed upper outer portion of the deltoid muscle when raising your arm outward (abduct).

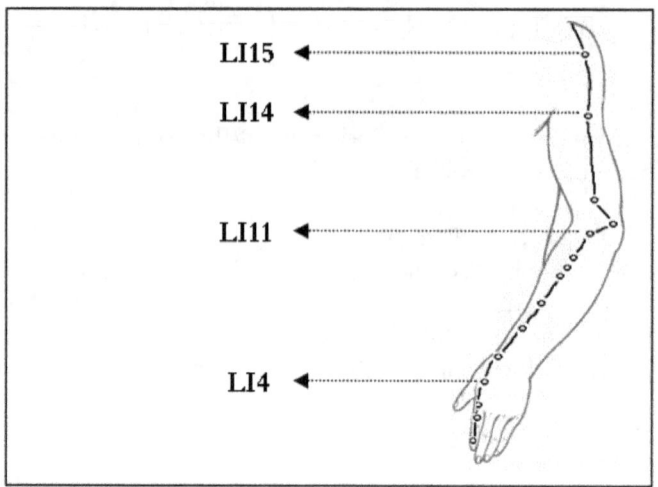

### GB21:

*Location:* It is situated at the highest point of the trapezius muscle, midway between the spinous process of C7 and the acromion process.

### TW2:

*Location:* It is situated 0.1 cun posterior to the ulnar side corner of the nail of the fourth finger.

### *TW5:*

*Location:* It is situated on the posterior side of the forearm, between the radius and the ulna, 2 cun above TW4.

### *TW6:*

*Location:* It is situated on the posterior side of the forearm, between the radius and the ulna, 3 cun above TW4.

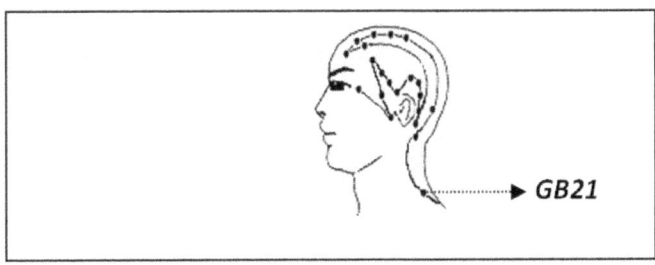

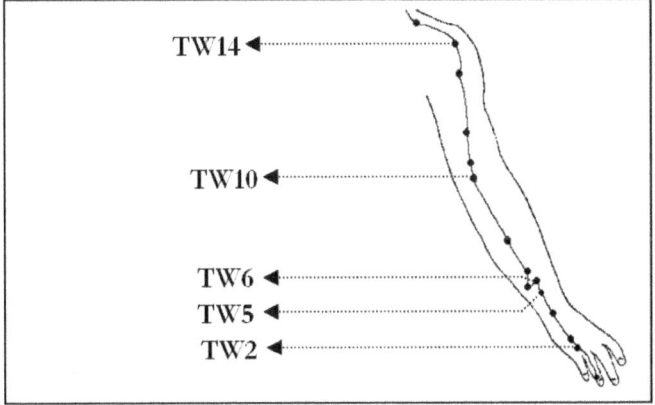

### *TW10:*

*Location:* It is situated in a depression formed with the elbow flexed, 1 cun superior to the olecranon.

### *TW14:*

*Location:* It is situated in the depression posterior and

inferior to the acromion process, about 1 cun posterior to LI15.

### SI5:
*Location:* It is situated in a depression near the ulnar end of the transverse wrist crease on the posterior side of the hand.

### SI6:
*Location:* It is situated in the bony cleft on the inner side of the wrist bone (ulnar tuberosity) on the dorsal side of the wrist.

### SI9:
*Location:* It is situated 1 cun above the posterior end of the axillary fold.

### SI10:
*Location:* It is situated in a depression inferior to spine of the scapula, straight above SI9.

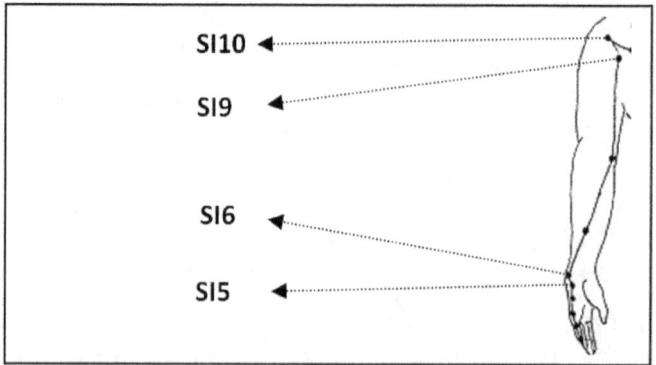

### HT3:
*Location:* It is situated at the medial end of the transverse

cubital crease (With elbow flexed).

### *HT7:*
*Location:* It is situated in the small depression between the pisiform and ulna bones, on the anteromedial side of the transverse crease of the wrist with the palm facing up.

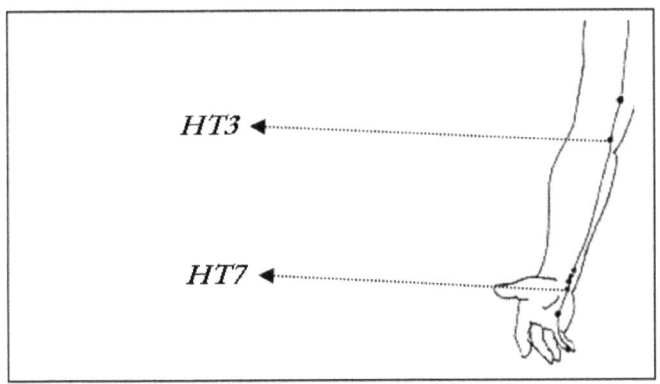

### *LU2:*
*Location:* Draw an imaginary line in the middle of your body between the chest. Go 6 cun outward. You'll find it 1 cun above the LU1.

### *LU5:*
*Location:* You can find it in the anterior fold of your elbow(cubital crease). Palpate the tendon (biceps brachii tendon) in the middle of it and then go outwards to locate the point.

### *LU9:*
*Location:* It is situated on the transverse crease of the wrist. Go outwards from the place we feel the pulse.

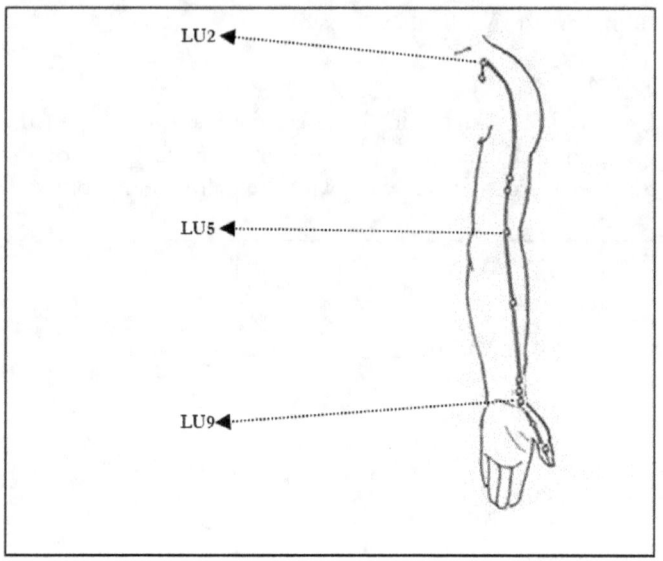

## P6:

*Location:* It is situated 2 cun above the the middle point (P7) of the transverse crease of the wrist between palmaris longus and flexor carpi radialis tendons.

## P7:

*Location:* It is situated in the middle of the transverse crease of the wrist between palmaris longus and flexor carpi radialis tendons.

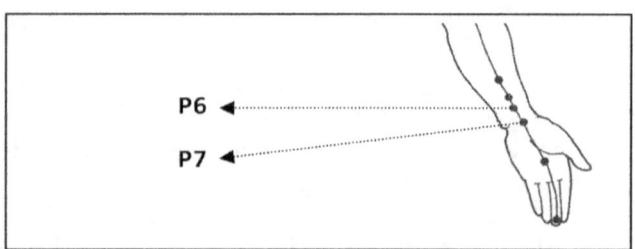

### *ST36:*

*Location:* It is situated 3 cun below ST35 slightly lateral to the anterior crest of the tibia.

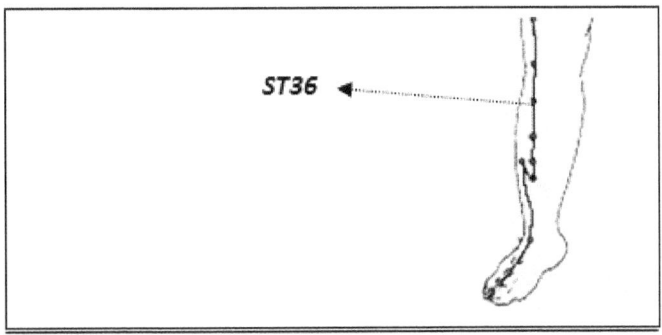

### *GV20:*

*Location:* It is situated midway on a line connecting the apex of both ears, 5 cun above midpoint of anterior hairline, and 7 cun above the midpoint of the posterior hairline.

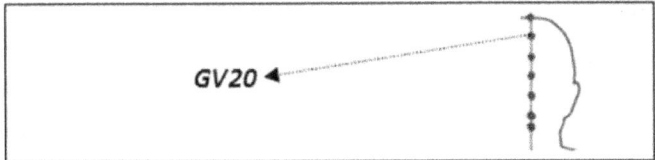

### *GB34:*

*Location:* It is situated in a depression anterior and inferior to the head of the fibula.

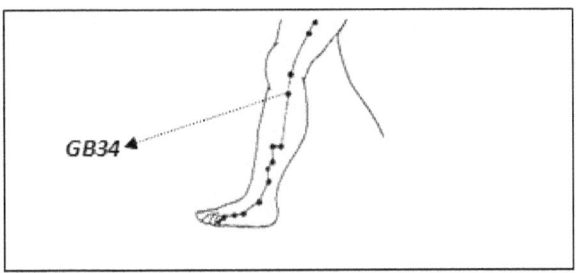

## *ii) Lower Limb Paresis / Paralysis*

### LU9:

*Location:* It is situated on the transverse crease of the wrist. Go outwards from the place we feel the pulse.

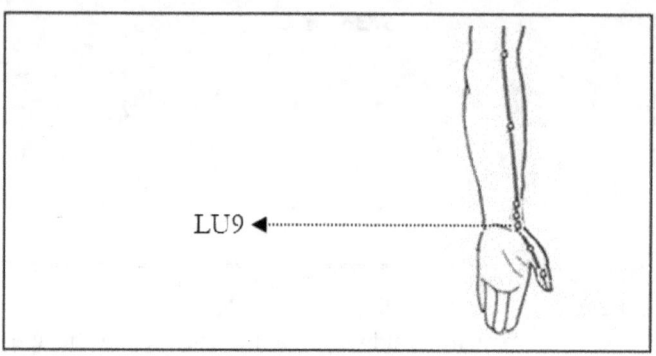

### BL36:

*Location:* It is situated on the spinal border of the scapula, 3 cun lateral to the body midline at the level of the spinous process of T2.

### BL37:

*Location:* It is situated on the spinal border of the scapula, 3 cun lateral to the body midline at the level of the spinous process of T3.

### BL40:

*Location:* It is situated 3 cun lateral the body midline at the level of the spinous process of T6.

### BL57:

*Location:* It is situated in a depression below the gastrocnemius muscle, 8 cun below to BL54.

### BL62:

*Location:* It is situated in a depression below the lateral malleolus.

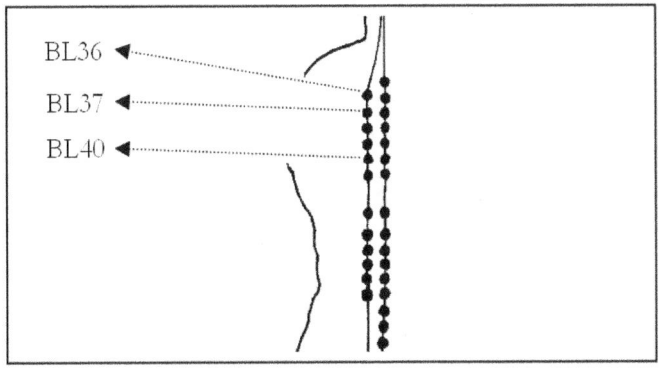

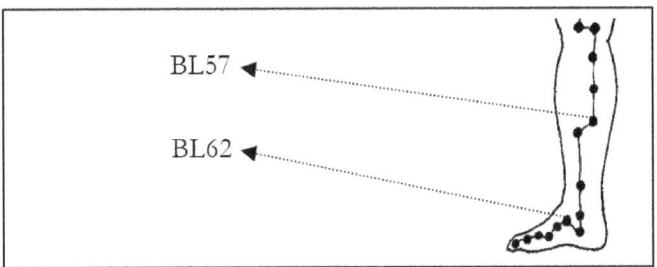

### *GB31:*

*Location:* It is situated on the lateral midline of thigh 7 cun above the transverse popliteal crease.

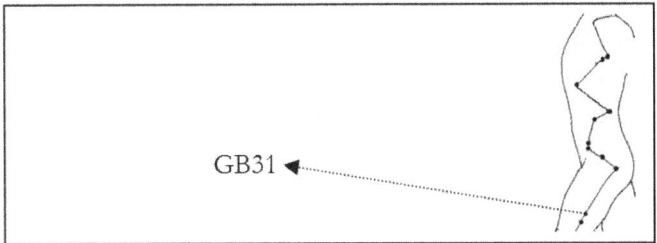

### GB34:

*Location:* It is situated in a depression anterior and inferior to the head of the fibula.

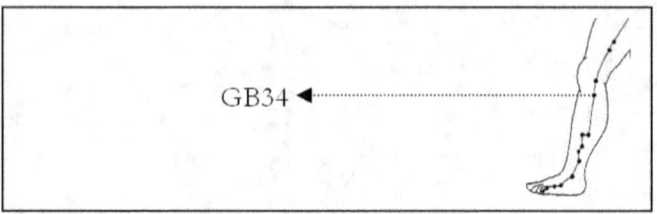

### GB39:

*Location:* It is situated in a depression between the posterior border of the fibula and the tendons of peroneous longus and brevis muscles, 3 cun above the tip of the outer anklebone (lateral malleolus).

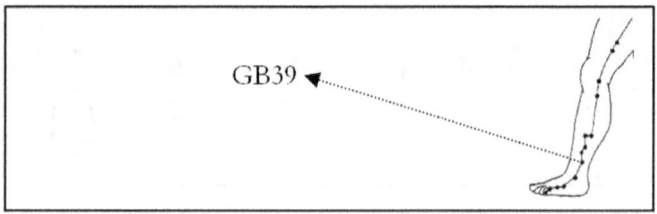

### ST31:

*Location:* It is situated straight below the anterior superior iliac spine (ASIS), in the depression lateral to the sartorius muscle.

### ST32:

*Location:* It is situated 6 cun above the superior outer border of the knee cap (patella bone) on the line connecting superior outer border of the knee cap (patella bone) and the ASIS.

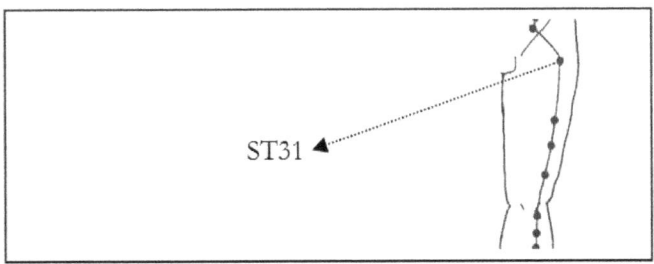

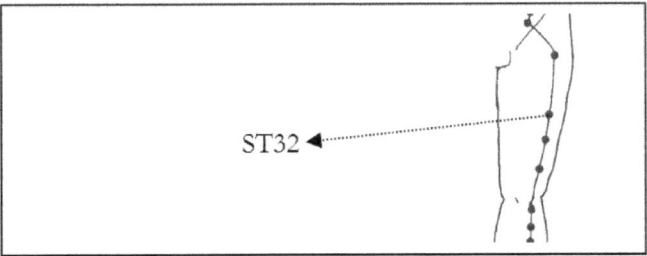

### *ST36:*

*Location:* It is situated 3 cun below ST35 slightly lateral to the anterior crest of the tibia.

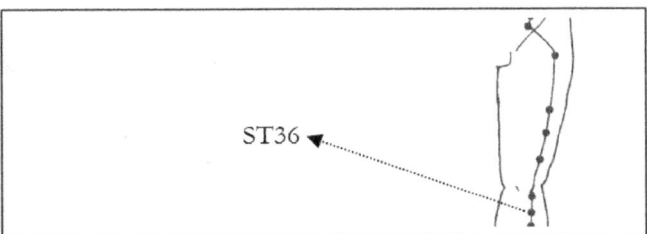

### *ST40:*

*Location:* It is situated one finger width lateral to ST38, 8 cun superior to the tip of the external malleous.

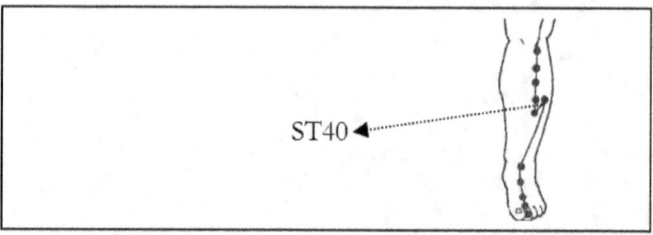

### *ST41:*
*Location:* It is situated at the midpoint of the transverse crease of the ankle joint on the dorsum of the foot, almost at the at the level of the tip of the outer anklebone (lateral malleolus).

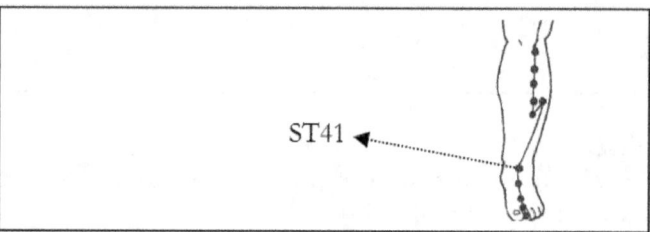

### *ST44:*
*Location:* It is situated in the depression distal and outer to the 2nd metatarsophalangeal joint, between the bases of the 2nd and 3rd toes.

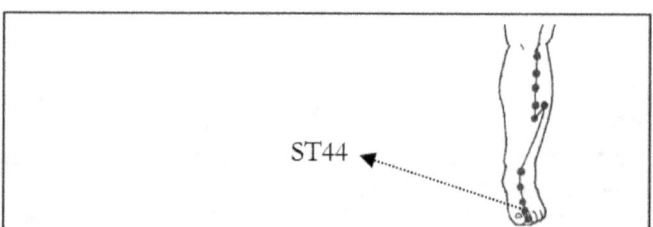

### SP6:

*Location:* It is situated 3 cun straight above the tip of the inner anklebone (medial malleolus).

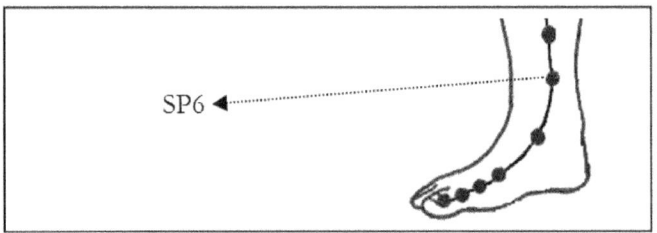

### SP9:

*Location:* It is situated in the depression between the posterior border of the tibia and gastrocnemius muscle on the lower border of the medial condyle of the tibia.

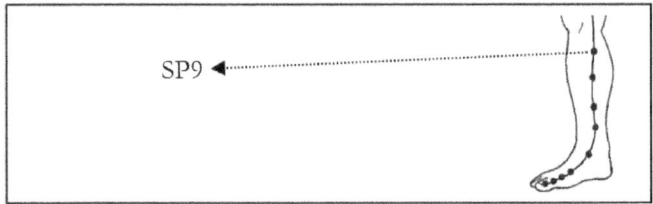

### KI3:

*Location:* It is situated at the level of the tip of the medial malleolus, in depression midway between the tip of the medial malleolus and the attachment of the Achilles tendon.

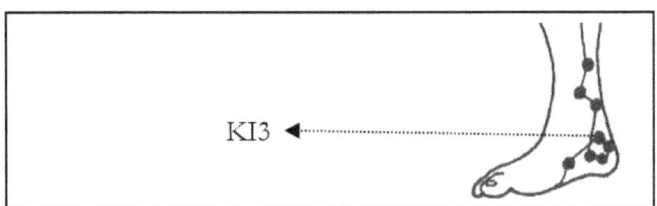

### KI5:

*Location:* It is situated in a depression anterior and superior to the medial tuberosity of the calcaneus, 1 cun directly below KI3.

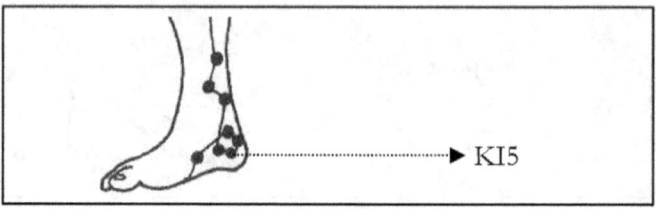

### LV6:

*Location:* It is situated 7 cun above the tip of the medial malleolus and posterior to the medial tibia.

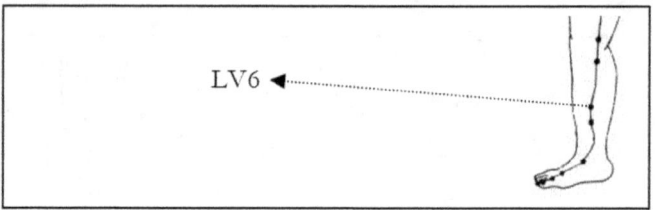

### LI4:

*Location:* It is situated between the 1st and 2nd metacarpal bones on the back side (dorsum) of the hand.

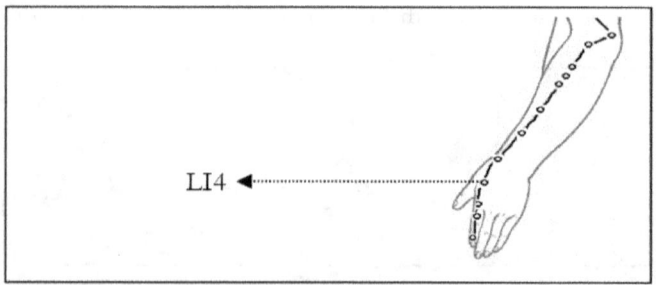

### *GV20:*

*Location:* It is situated midway on a line connecting the apex of both ears, 5 cun above midpoint of anterior hairline, and 7 cun above the midpoint of the posterior hairline.

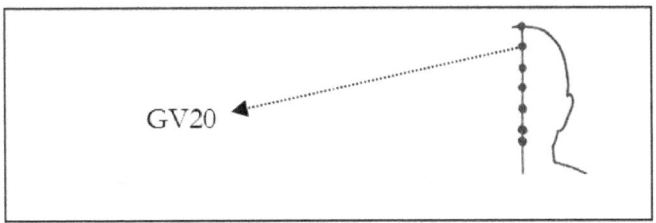

## b) Limbs' Weakness:

### *GB30:*

*Location:* It is situated at the junction of the lateral 1/3 and medial 2/3 of the distance between the greater trochanter and the hiatus of the sacrum.

### *GB31:*

*Location:* It is situated on the lateral midline of thigh 7 cun above the transverse popliteal crease.

### *GB34:*

*Location:* It is situated in a depression anterior and inferior to the head of the fibula.

### *GB43:*

*Location:* It is situated between the fourth and fifth metatarsals 0.5 cun proximal to the margin of the web on the dorsum of the foot.

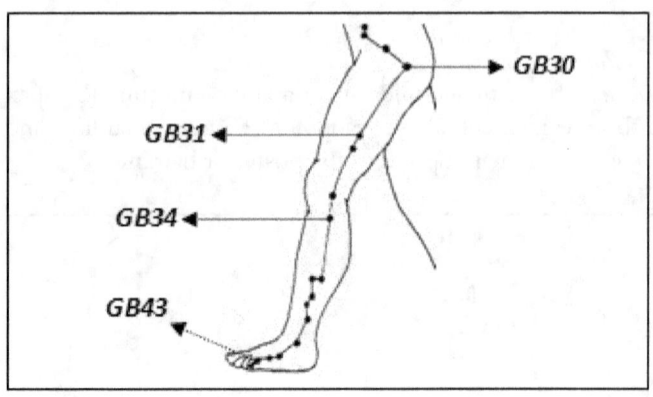

### BL20:
*Location:* It is situated 1.5 cun lateral to the body midline at the level of the spinous process of T11.

### BL25:
*Location:* It is situated 1.5 cun lateral to the body midline at the level of the spinous process of L4.

### BL28:
*Location:* It is situated 1.5 cun lateral to the body midline at the level of the second posterior sacral foramen.

### BL58:
*Location:* It is situated on the posterior border of the fibula, 7 cun above BL60, approx 1 cun lateral and inferior to BL57.

### BL61:
*Location:* It is situated below BL60, in a depression on the lateral calcaneus, posterior and inferior to the lateral malleolus.

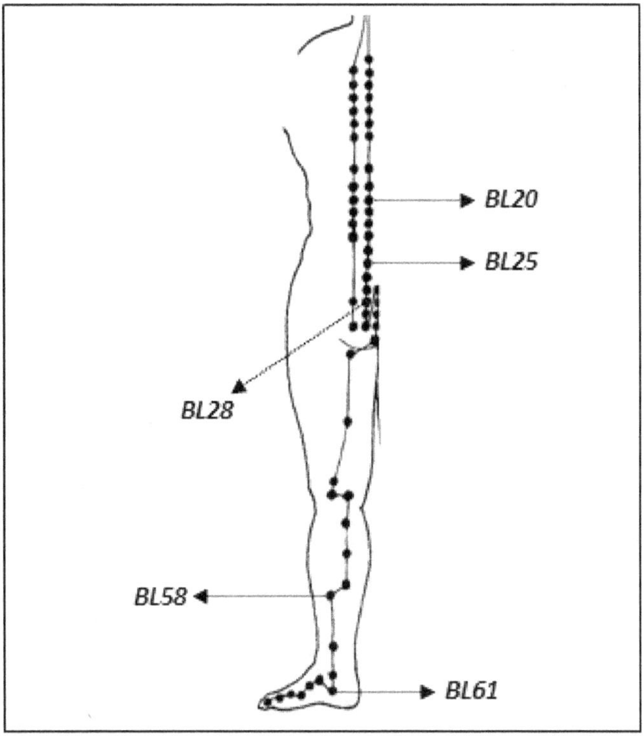

BL20
BL25
BL28
BL58
BL61

***CV6:***

*Location:* It is situated on the body midline, 1.5 cun inferior to the umbilicus.

CV6

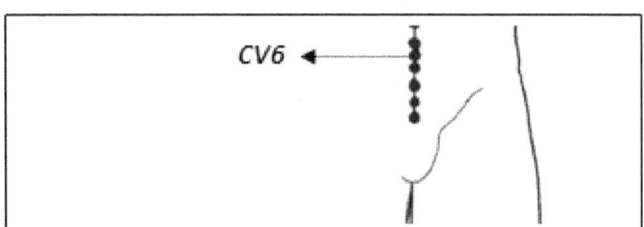

### KI3:

*Location:* It is situated at the level of the tip of the medial malleolus, in depression midway between the tip of the medial malleolus and the attachment of the Achilles tendon.

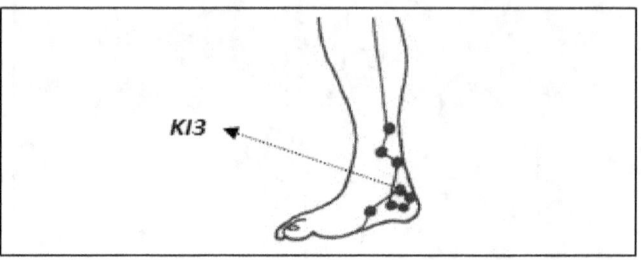

### LV13:

*Location:* It is situated on the lateral side of the abdomen below the free end of the 11th rib.

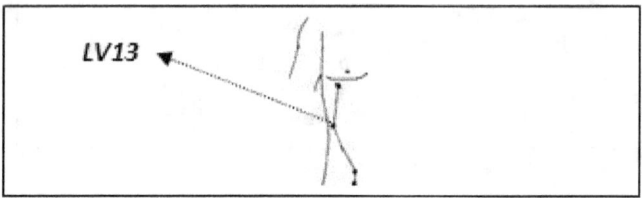

### P7:

*Location:* It is situated in the middle of the transverse crease of the wrist between palmaris longus and flexor carpi radialis tendons.

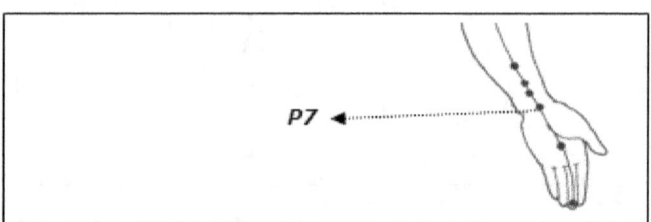

### SP7:

*Location:* is situated 6 cun from the tip of the inner anklebone (medial malleolus) or 3 cun above SP6.

### SP9:

*Location:* It is situated in the depression between the posterior border of the tibia and gastrocnemius muscle on the lower border of the medial condyle of the tibia.

### SP14:

*Location:* It is situated 4 cun lateral to the body midline, on lateral side of rectus abdominis muscle, 1.3 cun below the center of the umblicus.

### SP21:

*Location:* It is situated midway between the axilla and the anterior end of the 11th rib, on the midaxillary line, 6 cun inferior to the anterior axillary crease.

### ST31:

*Location:* It is situated straight below the anterior superior iliac spine (ASIS), in the depression lateral to the sartorius muscle.

### ST33:

*Location:* It is situated 3 cun above the superior outer border of the knee cap (patella bone) on the line connecting superior outer border of the knee cap (patella bone) and the ASIS.

### ST36:

*Location:* It is situated 3 cun below ST35 slightly lateral to the anterior crest of the tibia.

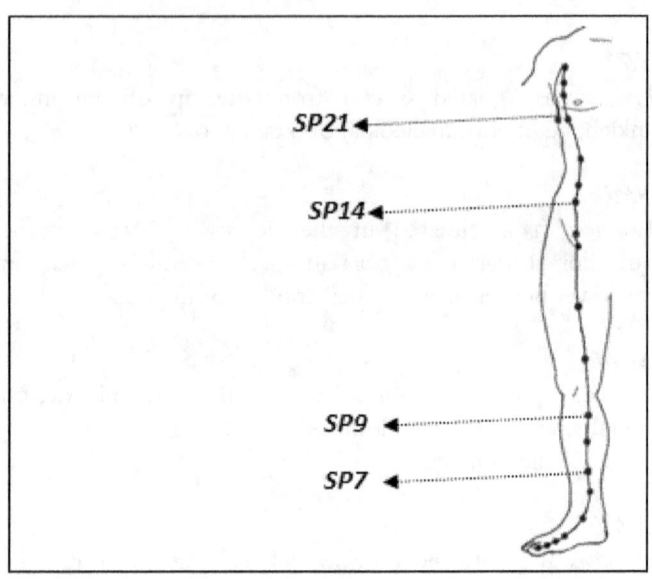

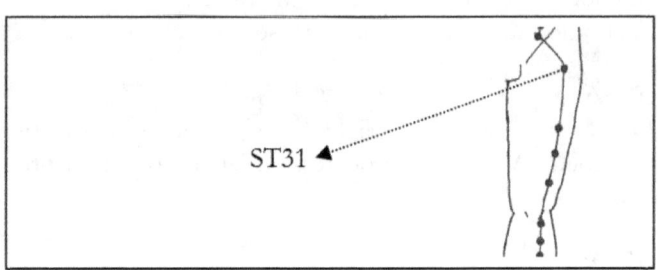

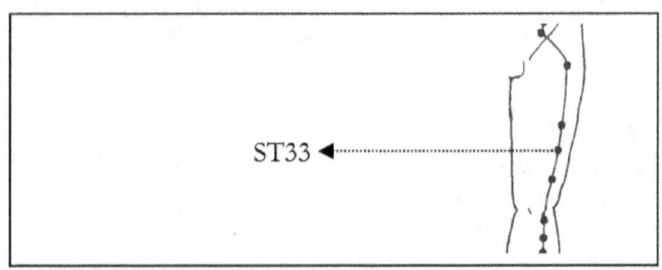

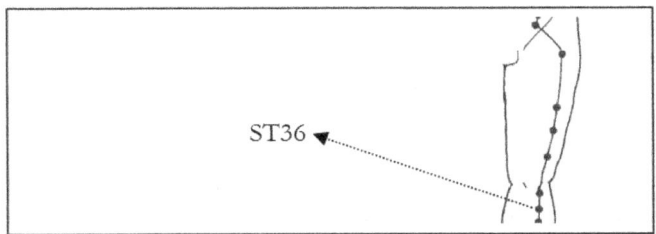

## c) Ataxia:

### *GB34:*

*Location:* It is situated in a depression anterior and inferior to the head of the fibula.

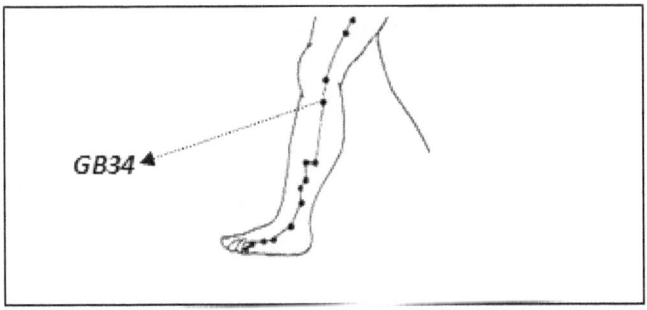

### *KI1:*

*Location:* It is situated in a depression on the sole of the foot (may be found when the foot is in plantar flexion) at the junction of the anterior 1/3 and posterior 2/3 of line connecting base of 2nd and 3rd toes and the heel.

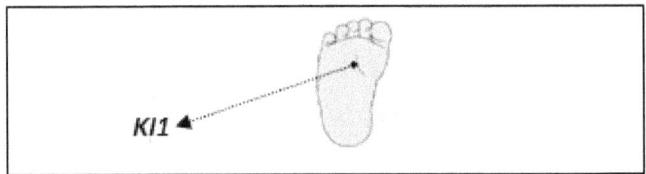

### *LI4:*

*Location:* It is situated between the 1st and 2nd metacarpal bones on the back side (dorsum) of the hand.

### *SI3:*

*Location:* It is situated in the depression proximal to the outer side of the 5th metacarpal bone (with a loose fist made).

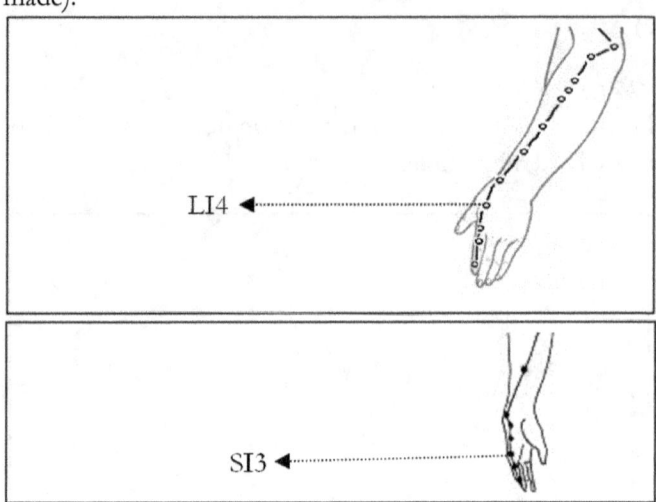

### *SI4:*

*Location:* It is situated in the depression between the fifth metacarpal bone and the hamate and pisiform bones, on the ulnar edge of the palm.

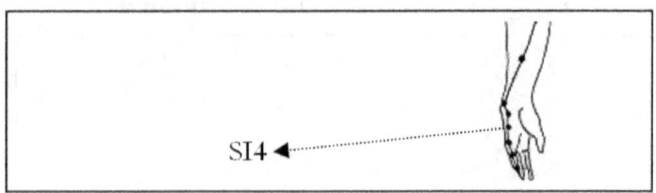

### *SP6:*

*Location:* It is situated 3 cun straight above the tip of the inner anklebone (medial malleolus).

### *ST36:*

*Location:* It is situated 3 cun below ST35 slightly lateral to the anterior crest of the tibia.

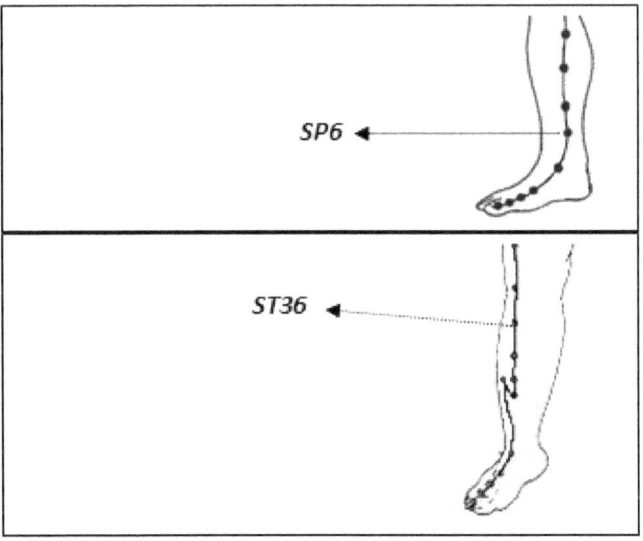

### *TW23:*

*Location:* It is situated in the depression at the lateral end of the eyebrow.

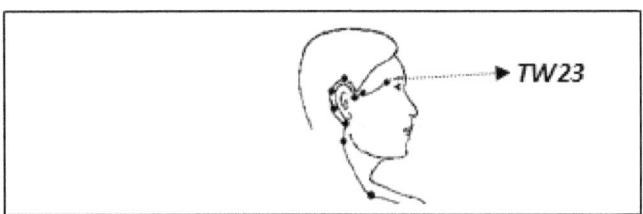

## d) Incoordination:

### *GB36:*

*Location:* It is situated 7 cun above the tip of the outer anklebone (lateral malleolus) on the anterior border of the fibula.

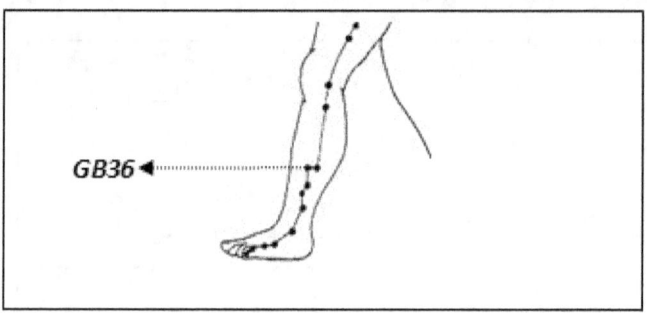

### *LI13:*

*Location:* It is situated 3 cun above LI11 on the line connecting LI11 and LI15 line.

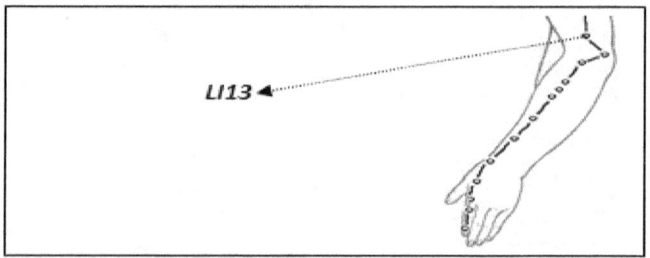

### *SI16:*

*Location:* It is situated on lateral side of neck, posterior to SCM, at the level of the adams apple.

## e) Difficulty in Speech:

### *BL38:*

*Location:* It is situated 3 cun lateral to the body midline at the level of the spinous process of T4.

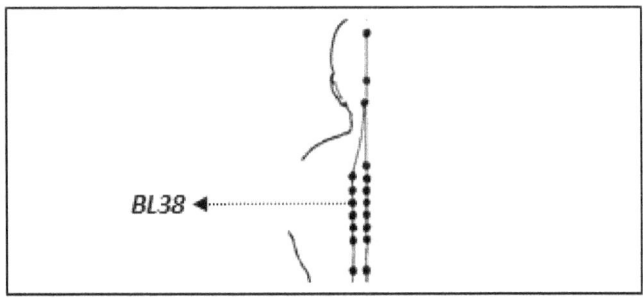

### *CV23:*

*Location:* It is situated on the body midline, in the depression superior to the hyoid bone.

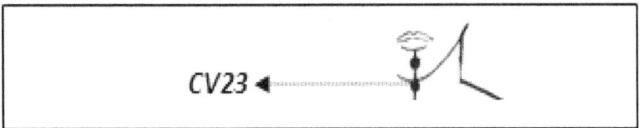

### *GV15:*

*Location:* It is situated in a depression below the spinous process of C1, 0.5 cun above the midpoint of the posterior hairline.

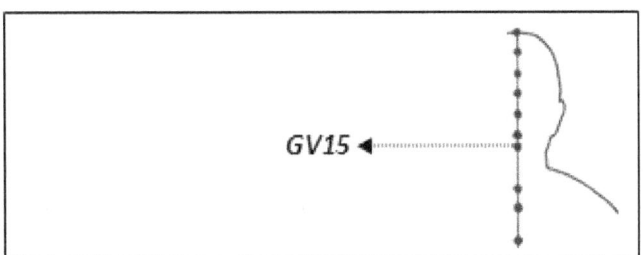

### GB20:
*Location:* It is situated in the depression created between the origins of the Sternocleidomastoid and Trapezius muscles, at the junction of the occipital and nuchal regions, lateral to the body midline.

### GB21:
*Location:* It is situated at the highest point of the trapezius muscle, midway between the spinous process of C7 and the acromion process.

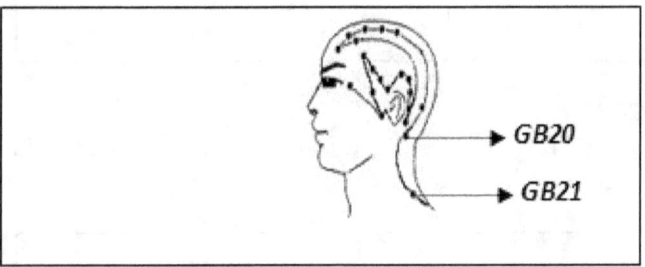

### KI1:
*Location:* It is situated in a depression on the sole of the foot (may be found when the foot is in plantar flexion) at the junction of the anterior 1/3 and posterior 2/3 of line connecting base of 2nd and 3rd toes and the heel.

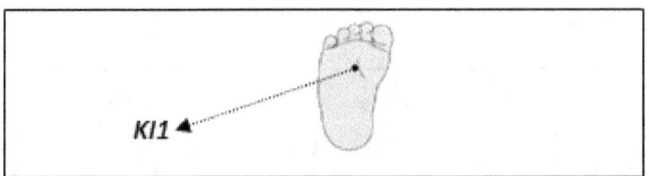

### LI4:
*Location:* It is situated between the 1st and 2nd metacarpal bones on the back side (dorsum) of the hand.

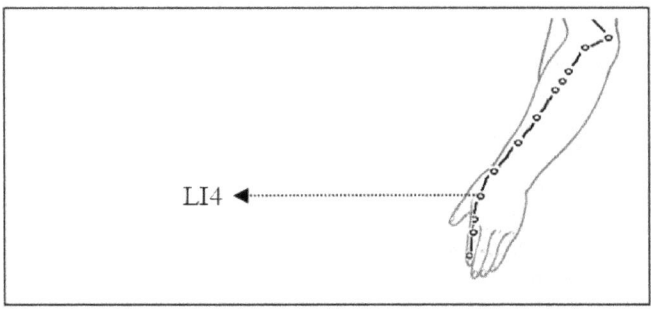

### *ST36:*

*Location:* It is situated 3 cun below ST35 slightly lateral to the anterior crest of the tibia.

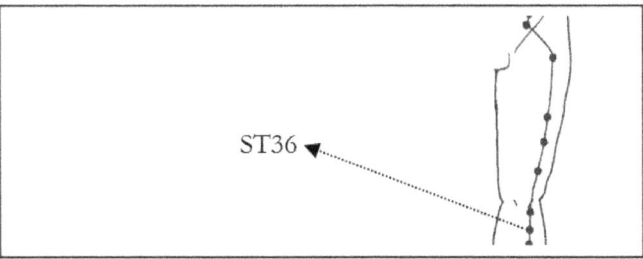

# 4 PSYCHOLOGICAL AND MENTAL PROBLEMS

The psychological and mental problems are common, mostly in the acute cases. Here we'll learn the acu points to get rid of mainly 5 problems:
 a)   Lack of Joy
 b)   Anxiety and Nervousness
 c)   Depression
 d)   Insomnia
 e)   Memory And Concentration

## a) Lack of Joy:

### *HT3:*
*Location:* It is situated at the medial end of the transverse cubital crease (With elbow flexed).

### *BL15:*
*Location:* It is situated 1.5 cun lateral to the body midline at the level of the spinous process of T5.

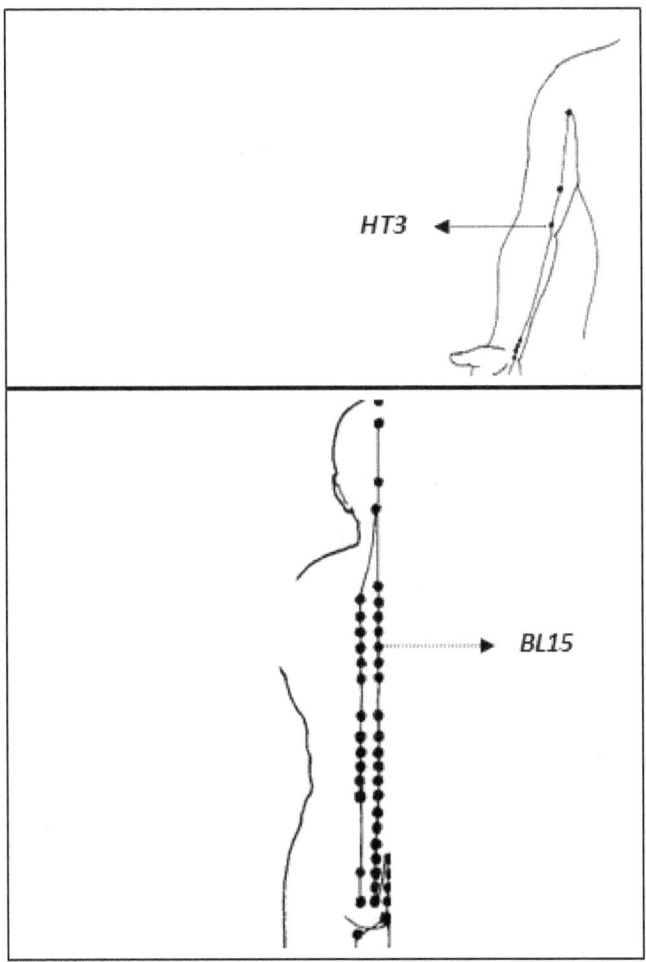

## b) Mental Emotional Component:

### GB20:

*Location:* It is situated in the depression created between the origins of the Sternocleidomastoid and Trapezius muscles, at the junction of the occipital and nuchal regions, lateral to the body midline.

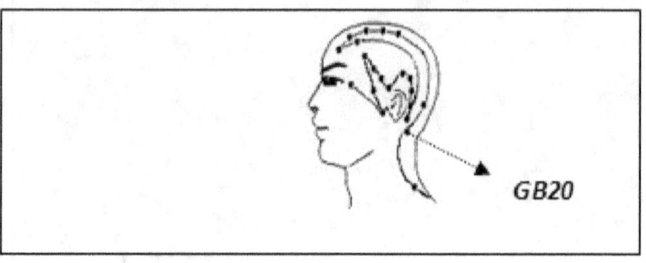

GB20

### c) Anxiety and Nervousness:

*P6:*

*Location:* It is situated 2 cun above the the middle point (P7) of the transverse crease of the wrist between palmaris longus and flexor carpi radialis tendons.

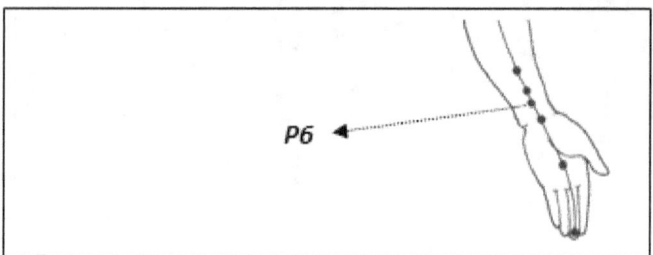

P6

*HT7:*

*Location:* It is situated in the small depression between the pisiform and ulna bones, on the anteromedial side of the transverse crease of the wrist with the palm facing up.

*TW15:*

*Location:* It is situated on the superior angle of the scapula midway between SI13 and GB21.

### *CV17:*

*Location:* It is situated on the body midline at the level of the 4th intercostal space.

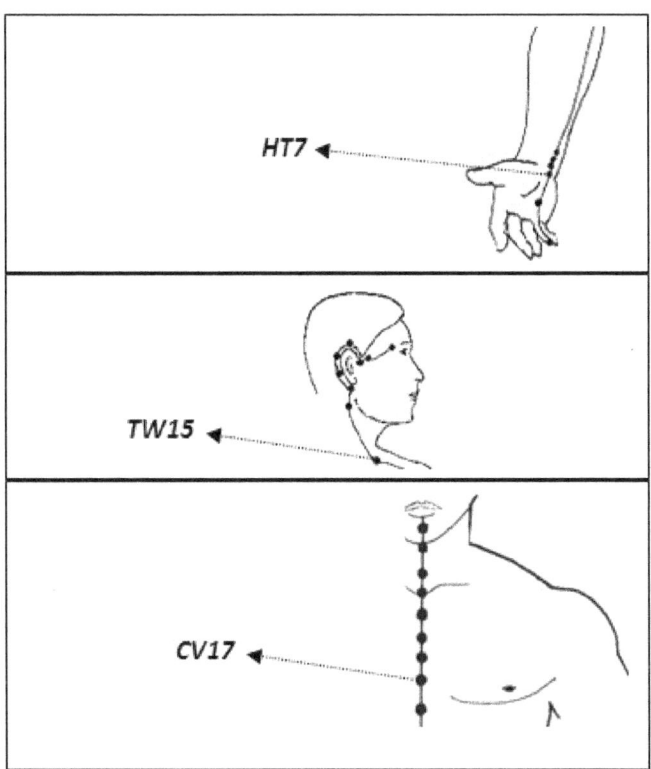

### d) Depression:

### *GV20:*

*Location:* It is situated midway on a line connecting the apex of both ears, 5 cun above midpoint of anterior hairline, and 7 cun above the midpoint of the posterior hairline.

### *GB20:*

*Location:* It is situated in the depression created between the origins of the Sternocleidomastoid and Trapezius muscles, at the junction of the occipital and nuchal regions, lateral to the body midline.

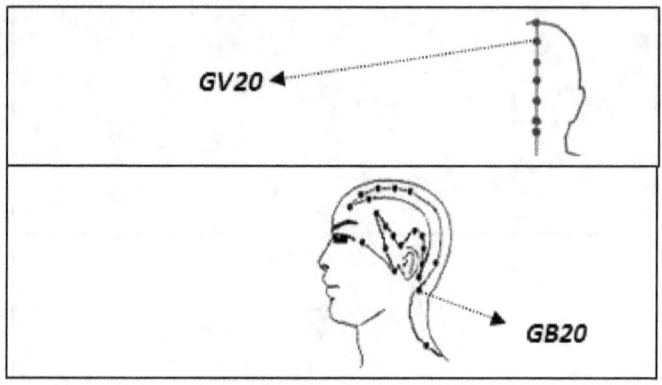

### TW15:

*Location:* It is situated on the superior angle of the scapula midway between SI13 and GB21.

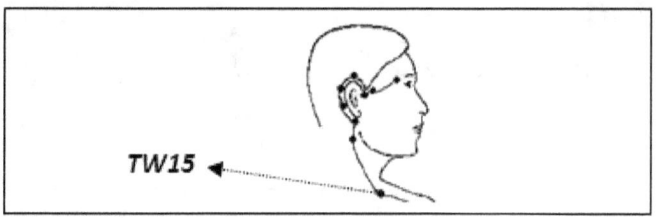

### KI27:

*Location:* It is situated in depression on lower border of clavicle, 2 cun lateral to the body midline.

### CV17:

*Location:* It is situated on the body midline at the level of the 4th intercostal space.

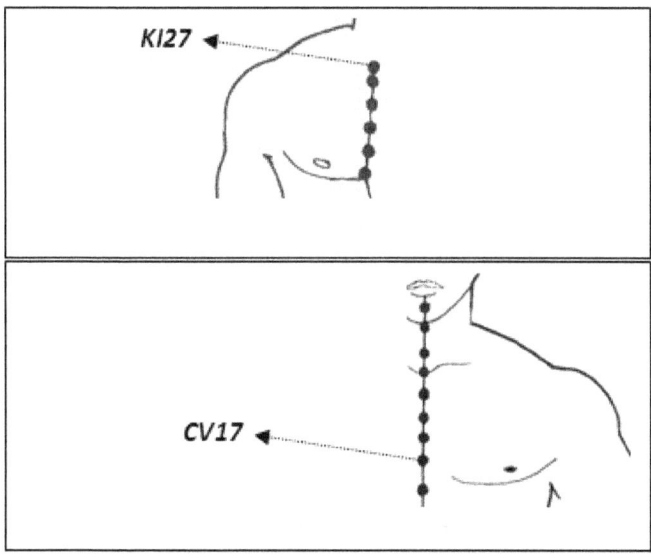

## *LU1:*

*Location:* Draw an imaginary line in the middle of your body between the chest. Go 6 cun outward to at the level of the 1st intercostal space.

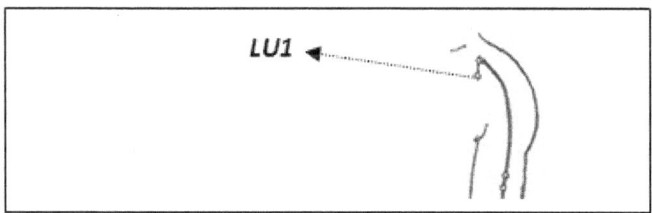

## *ST36: (forbidden for pregnant women)*

*Location:* It is situated 3 cun below ST35 slightly lateral to the anterior crest of the tibia.

## d) Insomnia:

### GB20:

*Location:* It is situated in the depression created between the origins of the Sternocleidomastoid and Trapezius muscles, at the junction of the occipital and nuchal regions, lateral to the body midline.

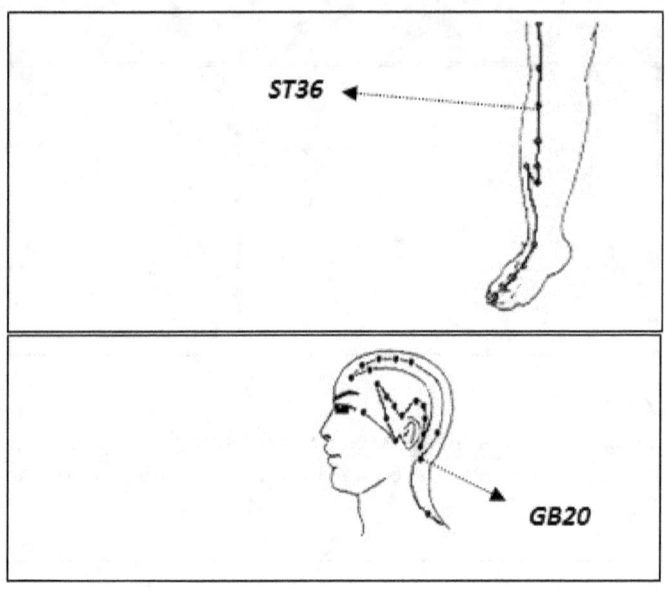

### GV16:

*Location:* It is situated in the depression between the trapezius muscles of both sides, below the external occipital protuberance, 1 cun above the midpoint of the posterior hairline.

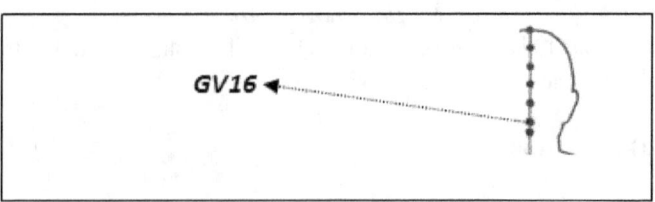

### *BL10:*

*Location:* It is situated in a depression on the lateral aspect of the trapezius muscle, 1.3 cun lateral to the body midline and 0.5 cun above the posterior hairline.

### *BL38:*

*Location:* It is situated 3 cun lateral to the body midline at the level of the spinous process of T4.

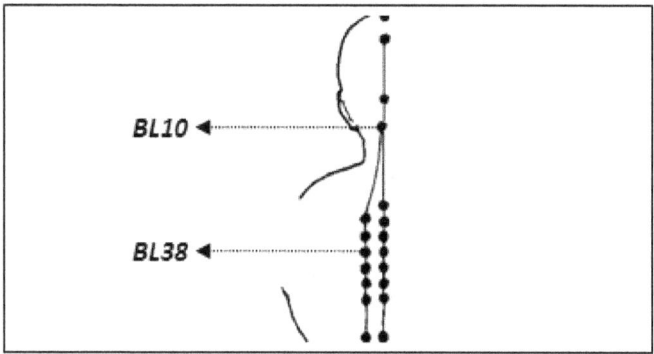

### *HT7:*

*Location:* It is situated in the small depression between the pisiform and ulna bones, on the anteromedial side of the transverse crease of the wrist with the palm facing up.

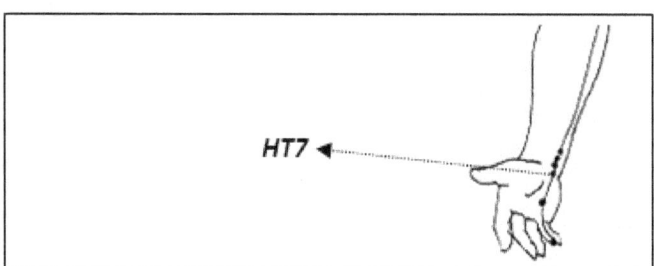

### KI3:
*Location:* It is situated at the level of the tip of the medial malleolus, in depression midway between the tip of the medial malleolus and the attachment of the Achilles tendon.

### KI6:
*Location:* It is situated in a depression 1 cun below the tip of the medial malleolus.

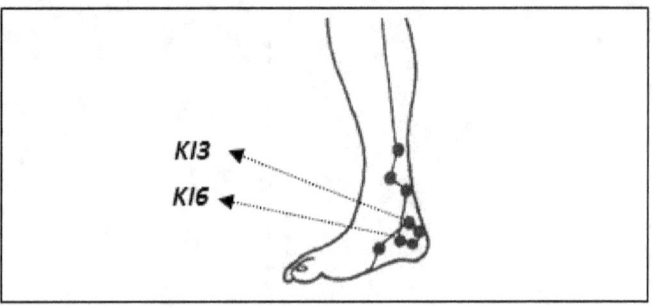

### SP6:
*Location:* It is situated 3 cun straight above the tip of the inner anklebone (medial malleolus).

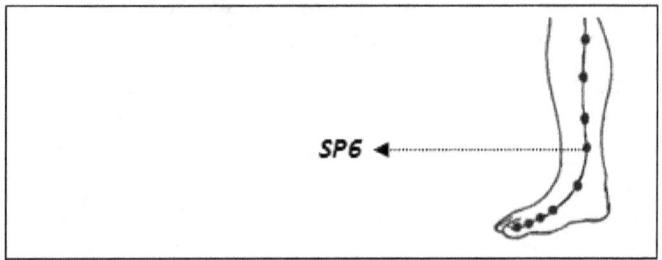

### CV17:
*Location:* It is situated on the body midline at the level of the 4th intercostal space.

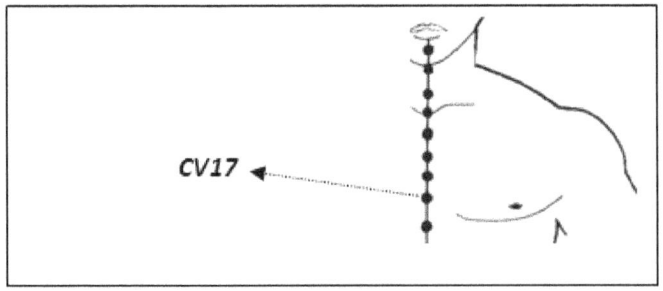

### e) Memory and Concentration:

#### *TW15:*

*Location:* It is situated on the superior angle of the scapula midway between SI13 and GB21.

#### *GB20:*

*Location:* It is situated in the depression created between the origins of the Sternocleidomastoid and Trapezius muscles, at the junction of the occipital and nuchal regions, lateral to the body midline.

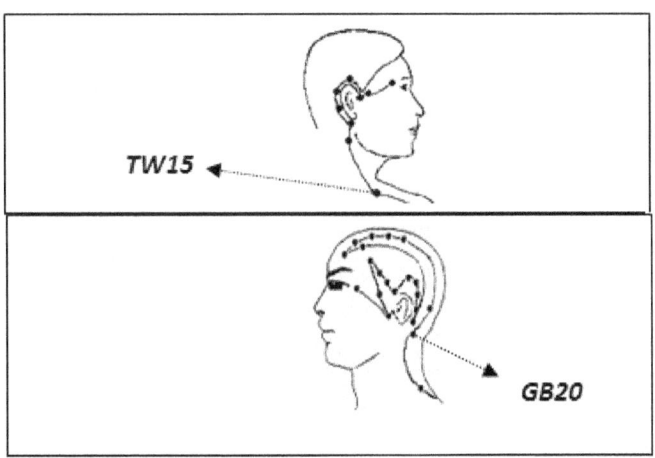

### GV26:

*Location:* It is situated at junction of the upper and middle third of philtrum.

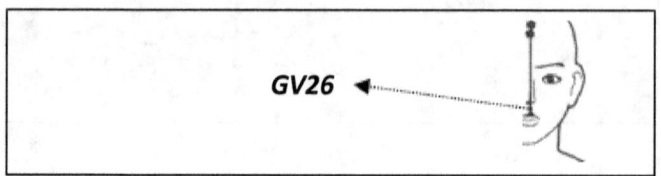

### CV17:

*Location:* It is situated on the body midline at the level of the 4th intercostal space.

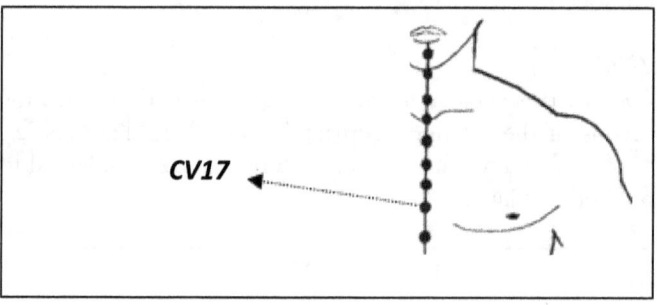

# 5 DIGESTIVE PROBLEM

The most common digestive problem in Muscular Dystrophy is *constipation*. The following points may help you.

### *BL25:*
*Location:* It is situated 1.5 cun lateral to the body midline at the level of the spinous process of L4.

### *BL27:*
*Location:* It is situated 1.5 cun lateral to the body midline at the level of the first posterior sacral foramen.

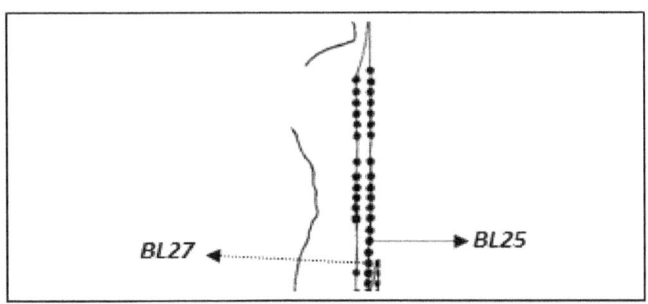

### CV6:
*Location:* It is situated on the body midline, 1.5 cun inferior to the umbilicus.

### CV12:
*Location:* It is situated on the body midline, 4 cun superior to the umbilicus.

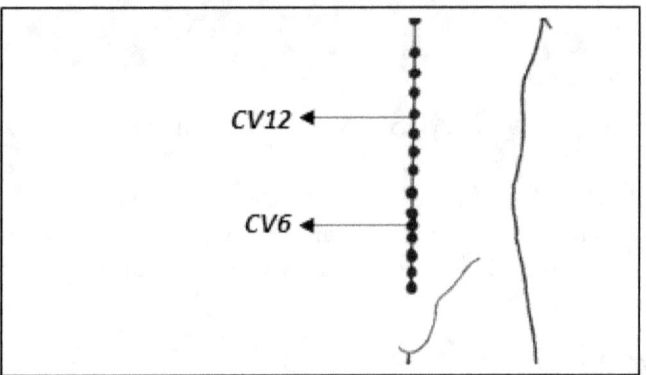

### SP15:
*Location:* It is situated 4 cun lateral to the body midline, on lateral side of rectus abdominis muscle, at the level of the center of the umblicus.

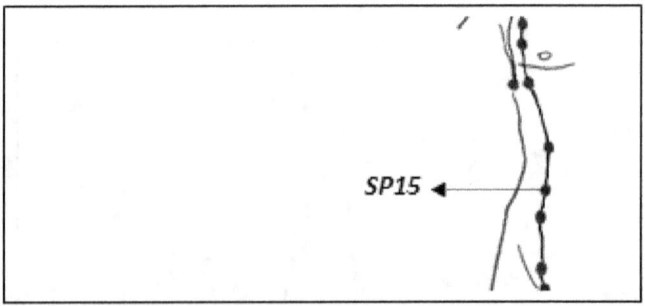

### *ST36:*

*Location:* It is situated 3 cun below ST35 slightly lateral to the anterior crest of the tibia.

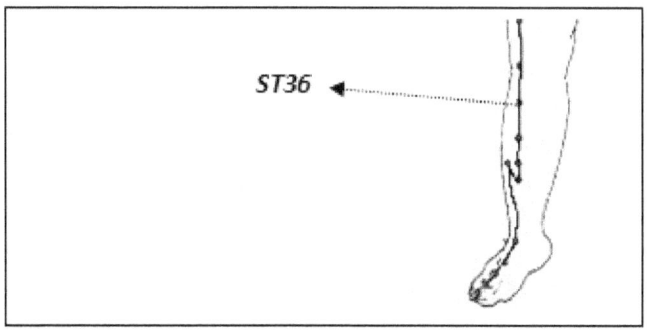

### *LV3:*

*Location:* It is situated in a depression distal to the junction of the 1st and 2nd metatarsal bones on dorsum of the foot.

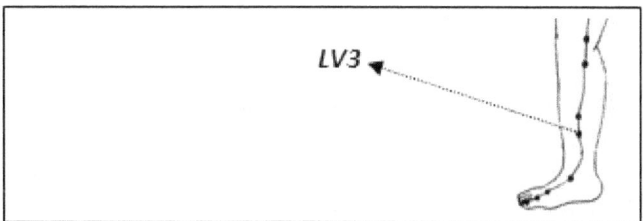

# 6 URINARY PROBLEMS

The two major urinary problems in the Muscular Dystrophy patients are *Loss of bladder control* and *urinary retention*.

## a) Loss of bladder control:

### *CV2:*
*Location:* It is situated on top of the notch in center of superior border of the pubic symphysis.

### *CV4:*
*Location:* It is situated on the body midline, 3 cun inferior to the umbilicus.

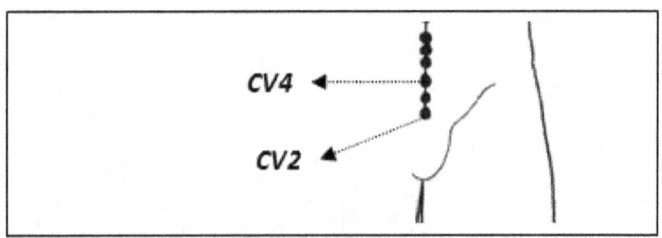

### *KI3:*

*Location:* It is situated at the level of the tip of the medial malleolus, in depression midway between the tip of the medial malleolus and the attachment of the Achilles tendon.

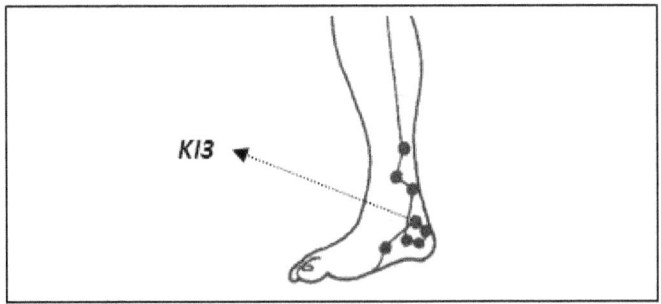

### *SP6:*

*Location:* It is situated 3 cun straight above the tip of the inner anklebone (medial malleolus).

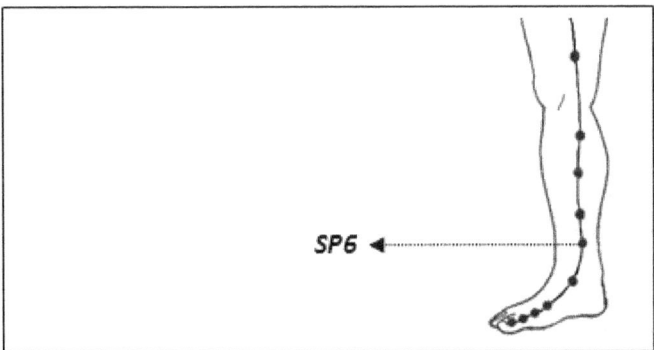

### *SI3:*

*Location:* It is situated in the depression proximal to the outer side of the 5th metacarpal bone (with a loose fist made).

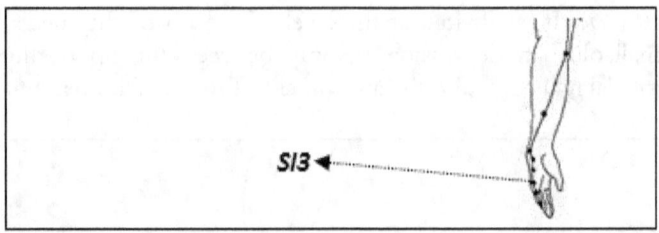

### *TW15:*
*Location:* It is situated on the superior angle of the scapula midway between SI13 and GB21.

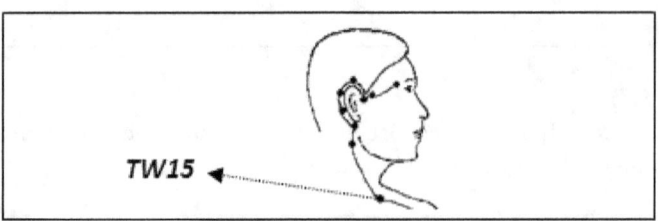

## b) Urinary Retention:

### *SP6:*
*Location:* It is situated 3 cun straight above the tip of the inner anklebone (medial malleolus).

### *SP9:*
*Location:* It is situated in the depression between the posterior border of the tibia and gastrocnemius muscle on the lower border of the medial condyle of the tibia.

### *TW15:*
*Location:* It is situated on the superior angle of the scapula midway between SI13 and GB21.

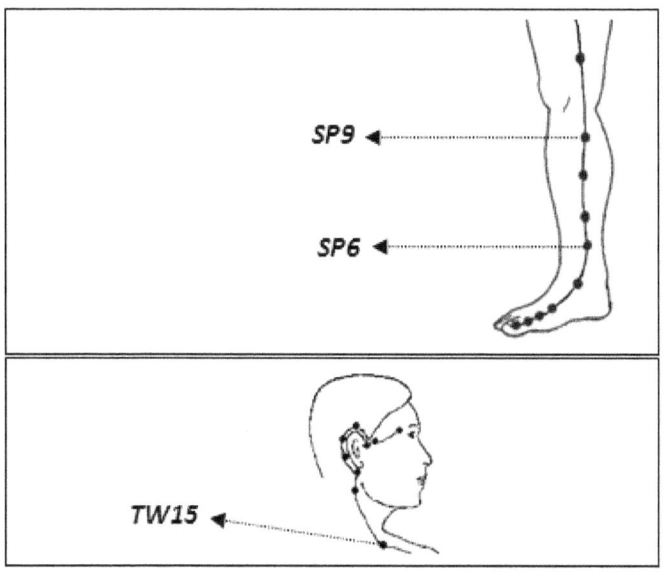

# 7 SEXUAL PROBLEMS

You may cop up with the sexual disability and loss of libido by administration pressure on the following points.

### *BL27:*
*Location:* It is situated 1.5 cun lateral to the body midline at the level of the first posterior sacral foramen.

### *BL34:*
*Location:* It is situated in the fourth posterior sacral foramen.

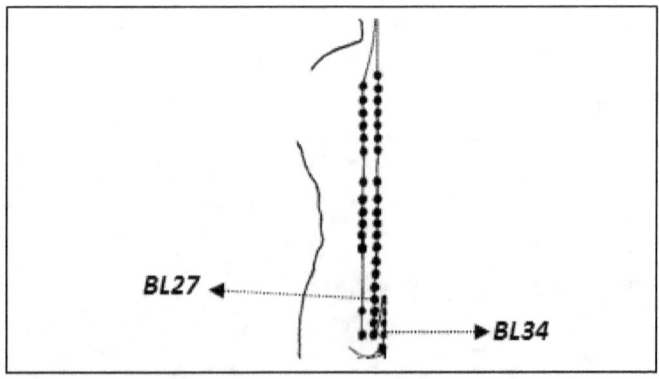

### *CV4:*

*Location:* It is situated on the body midline, 3 cun inferior to the umbilicus.

### *CV6:*

*Location:* It is situated on the body midline, 1.5 cun inferior to the umbilicus.

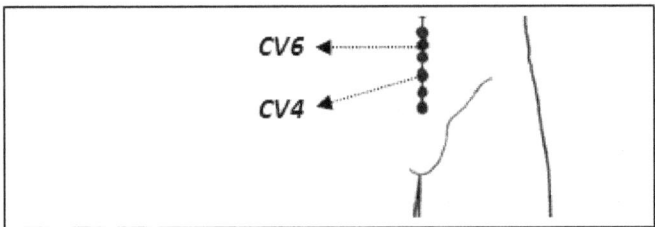

### *SP6 (forbidden for pregnant women):*

*Location:* It is situated 3 cun straight above the tip of the inner anklebone (medial malleolus).

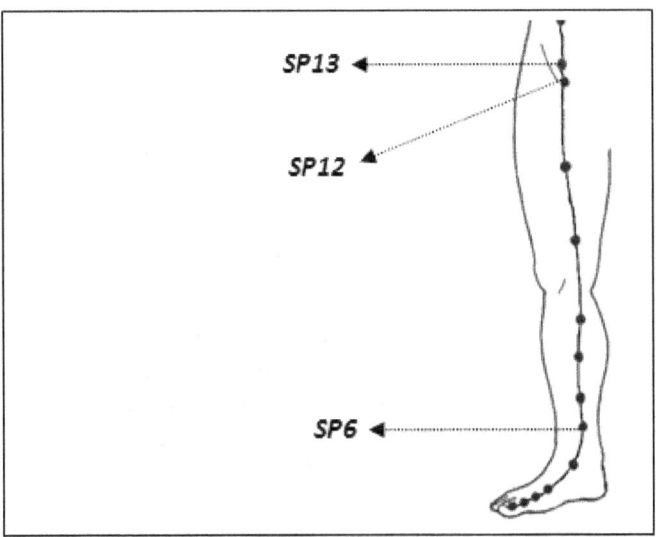

### SP12:

*Location:* It is situated in the inguinal region, 3.5 cun lateral to the body midline.

### SP13:

*Location:* It is situated 4 cun lateral to the body midline, 0.7 cun laterosuperior to SP12.

### ST36 (forbidden for pregnant women):

*Location:* It is situated 4 cun lateral to the body midline below ST12 on the line connecting the ST12 and the center of nipple, in the midpoint of the fossa below the clavicle bone.

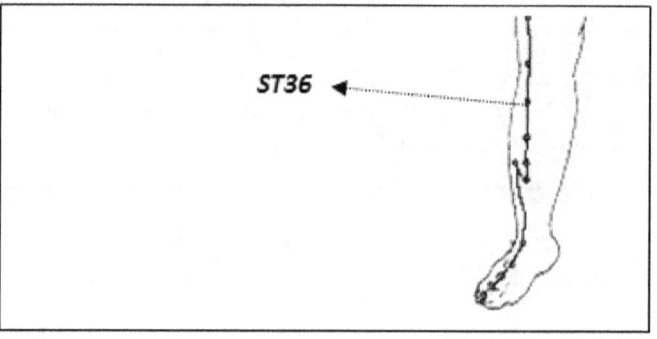

### GV4:

*Location:* It is situated below the spinous process of L2.

### KI1:

*Location:* It is situated in a depression on the sole of the foot (may be found when the foot is in plantar flexion) at the junction of the anterior 1/3 and posterior 2/3 of line connecting base of 2nd and 3rd toes and the heel.

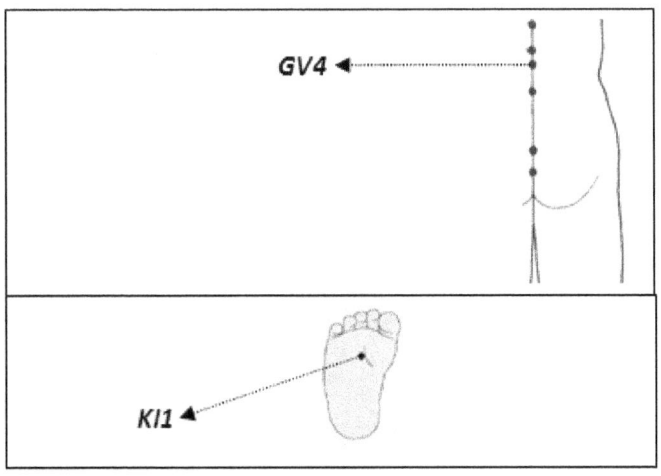

# APPENDIX

---

# CHARTS OF THE MEREDIANS

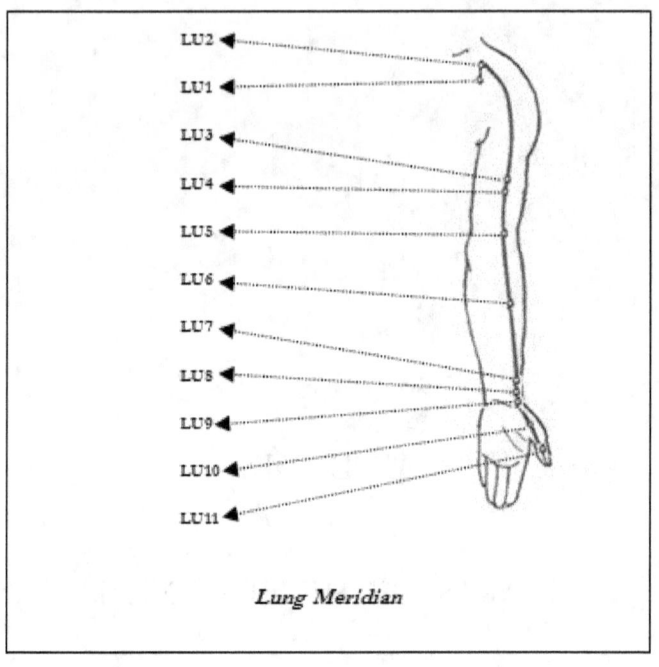

*Lung Meridian*

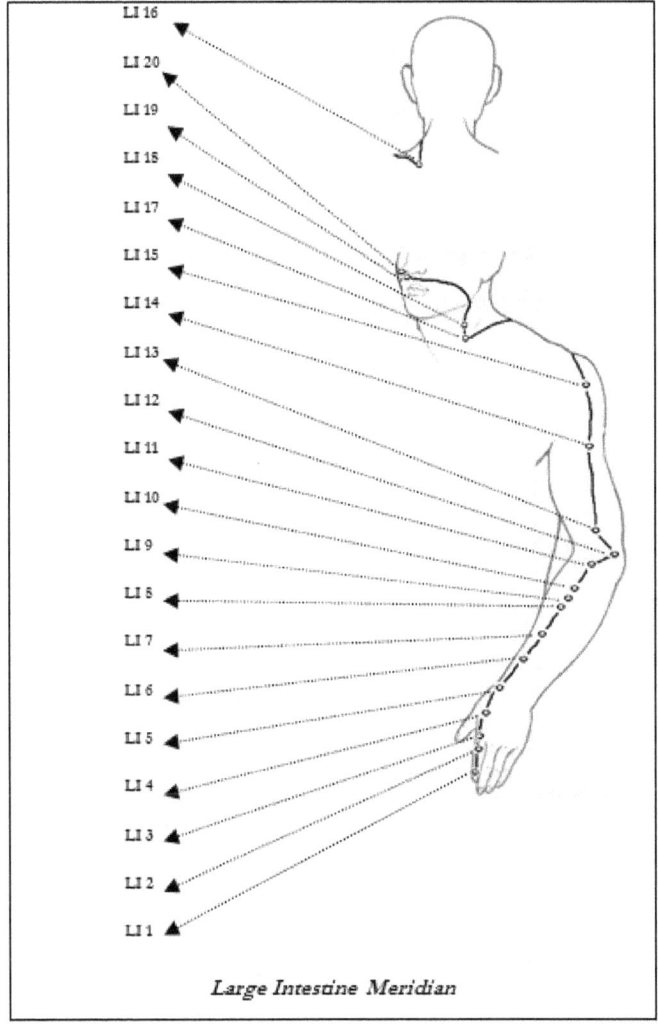

*Large Intestine Meridian*

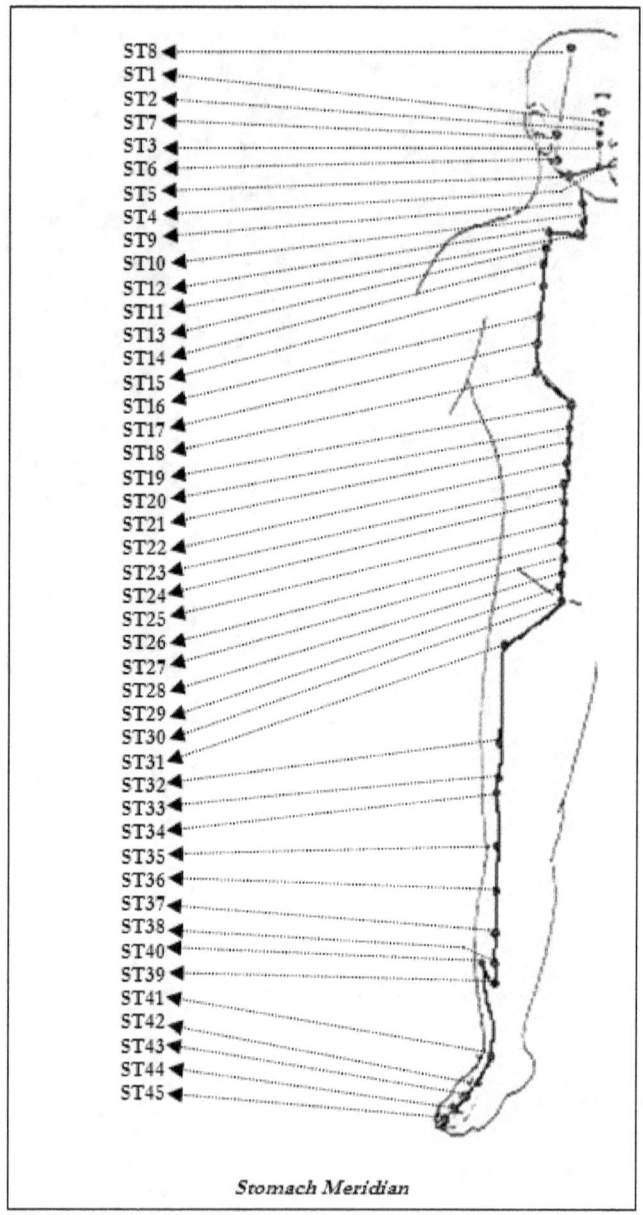

*Stomach Meridian*

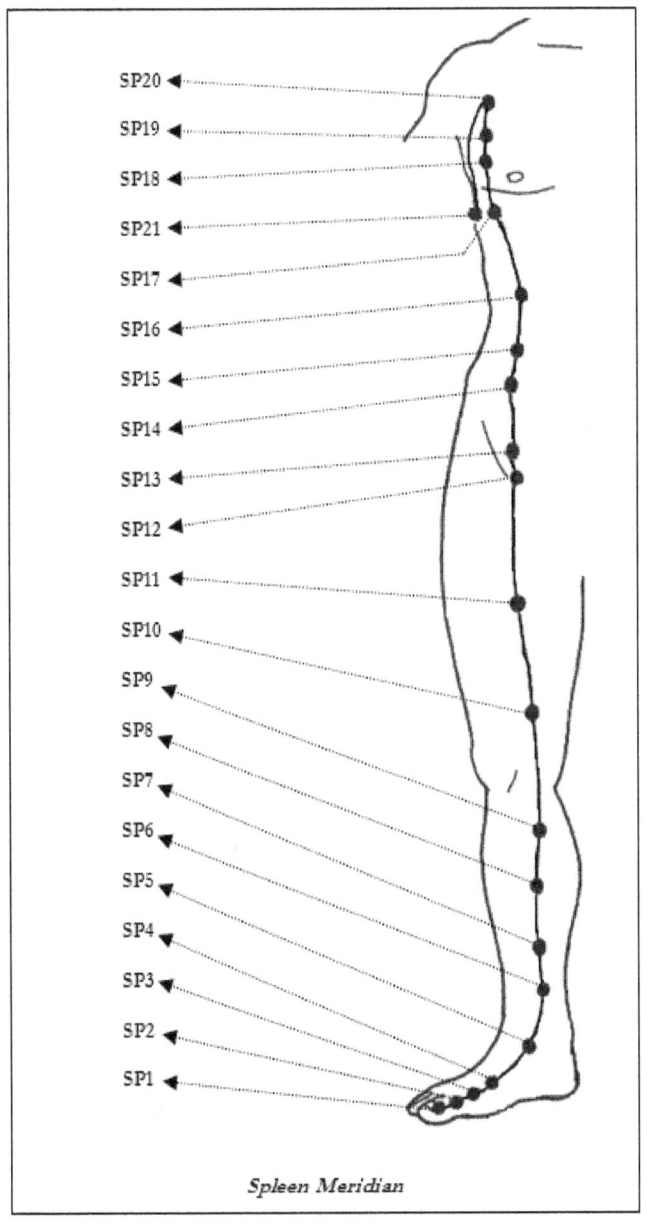

*Spleen Meridian*

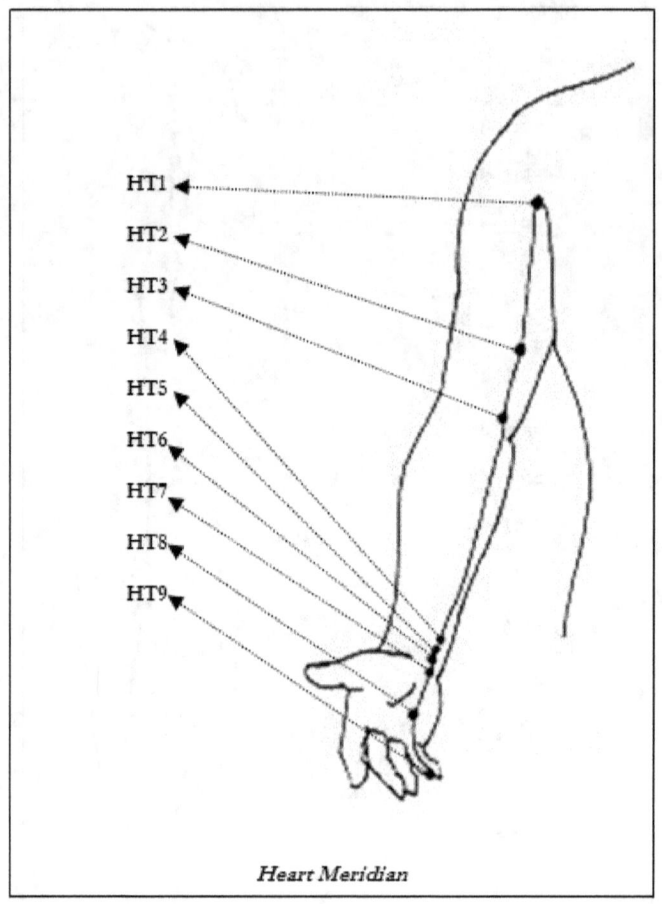

*Heart Meridian*

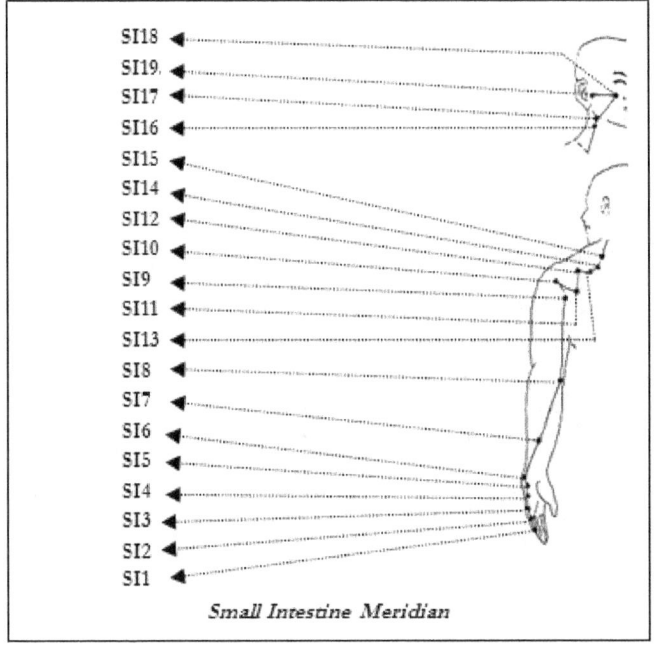

*Small Intestine Meridian*

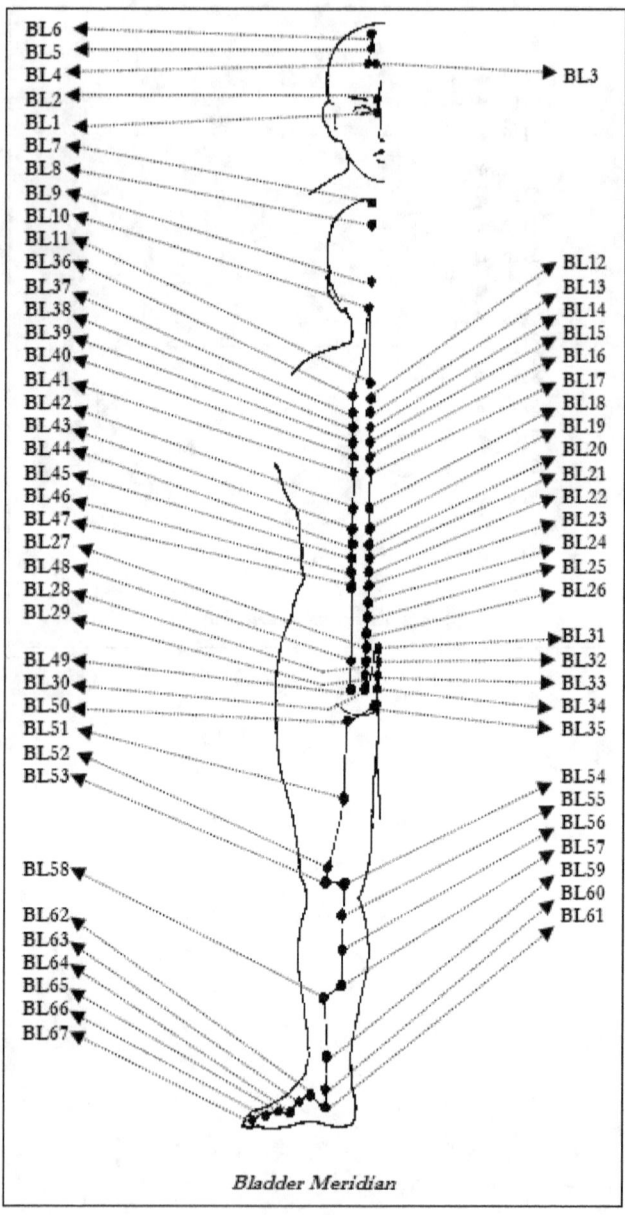

*Bladder Meridian*

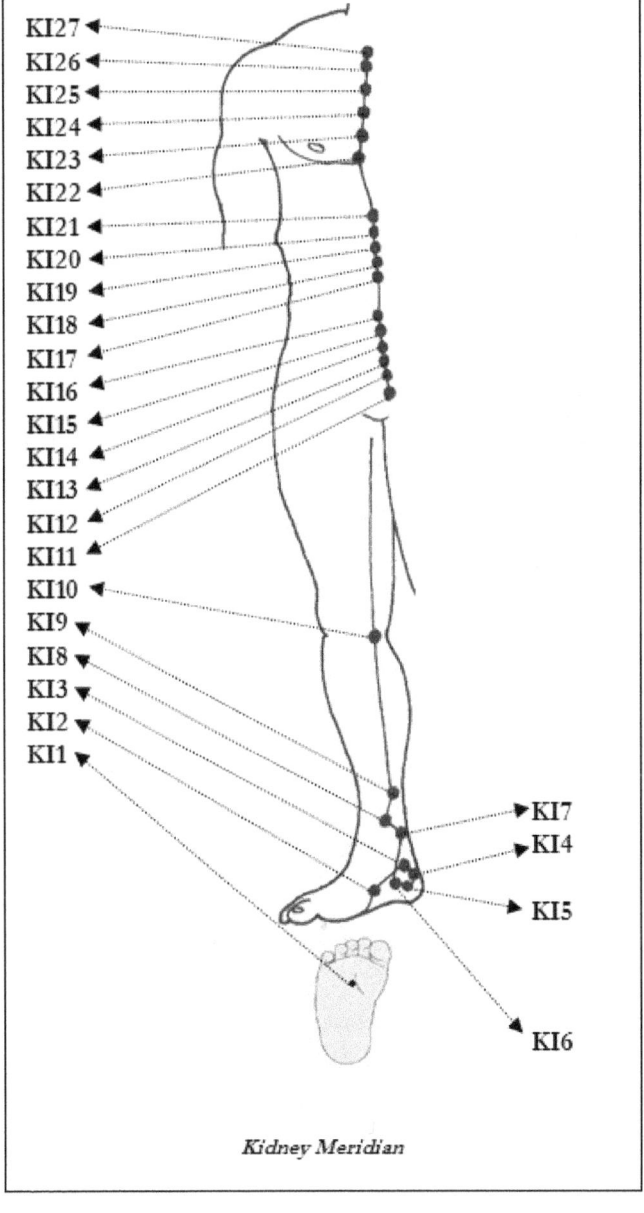

*Kidney Meridian*

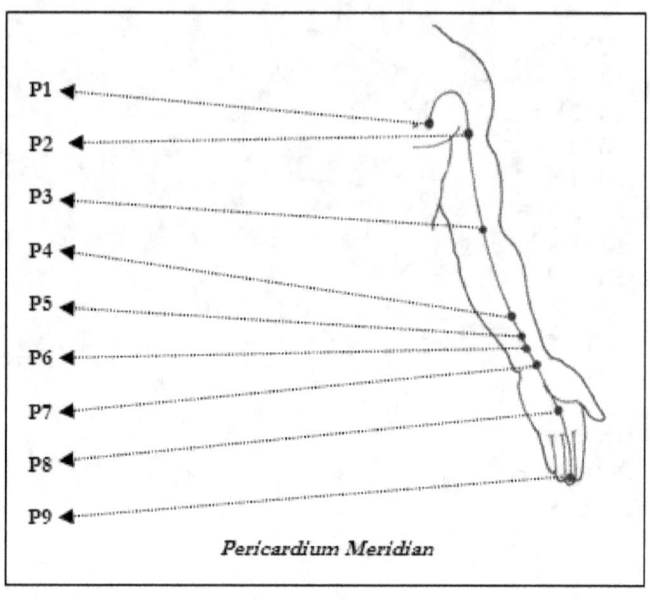

*Pericardium Meridian*

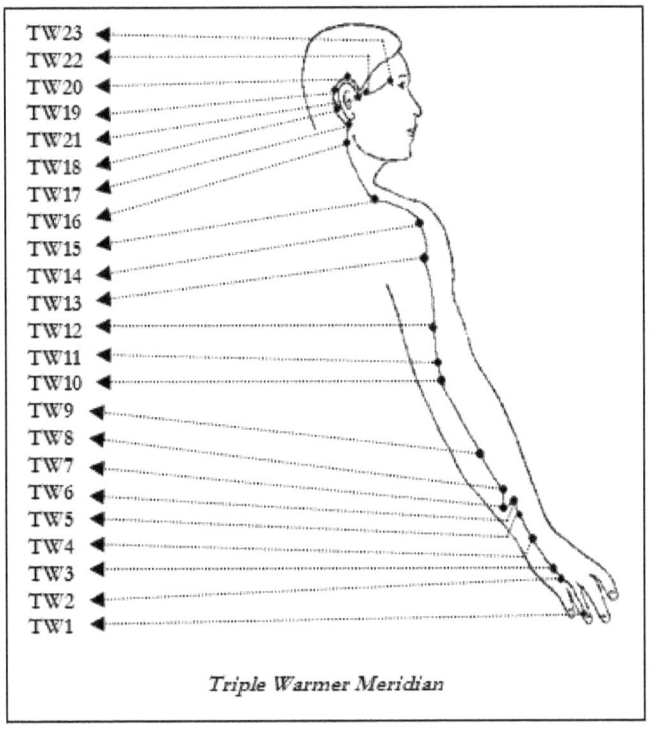

*Triple Warmer Meridian*

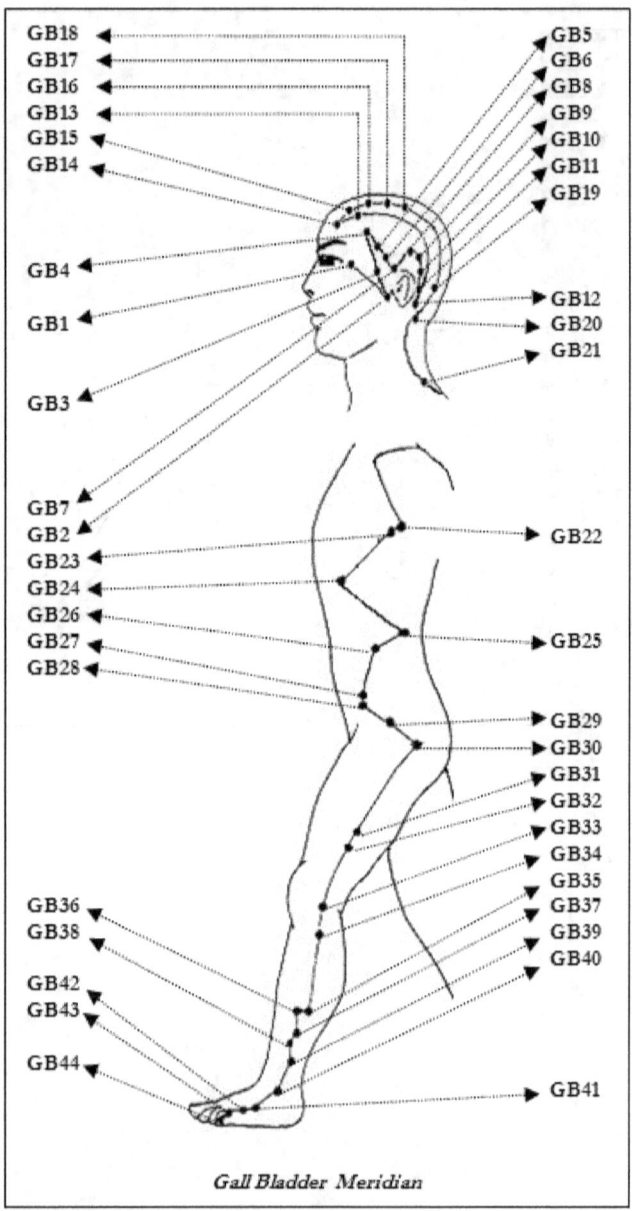

*Gall Bladder Meridian*

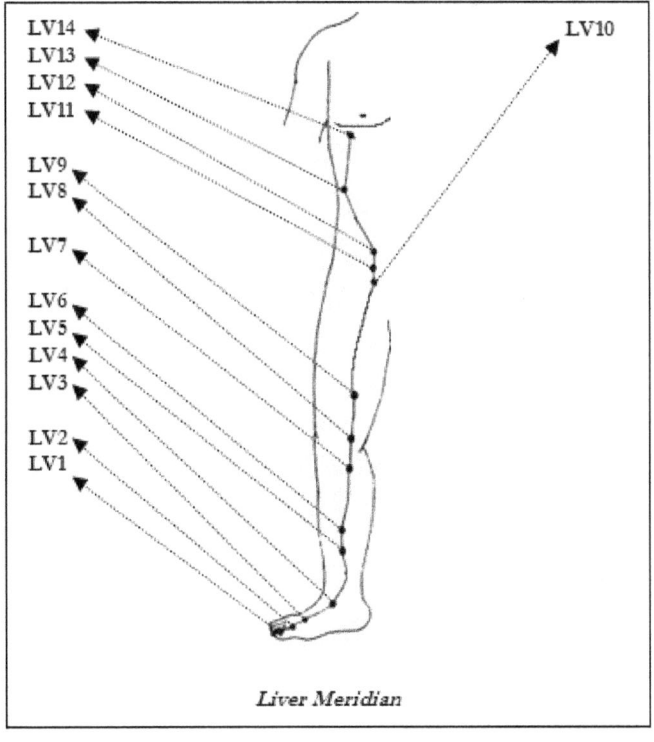

*Liver Meridian*

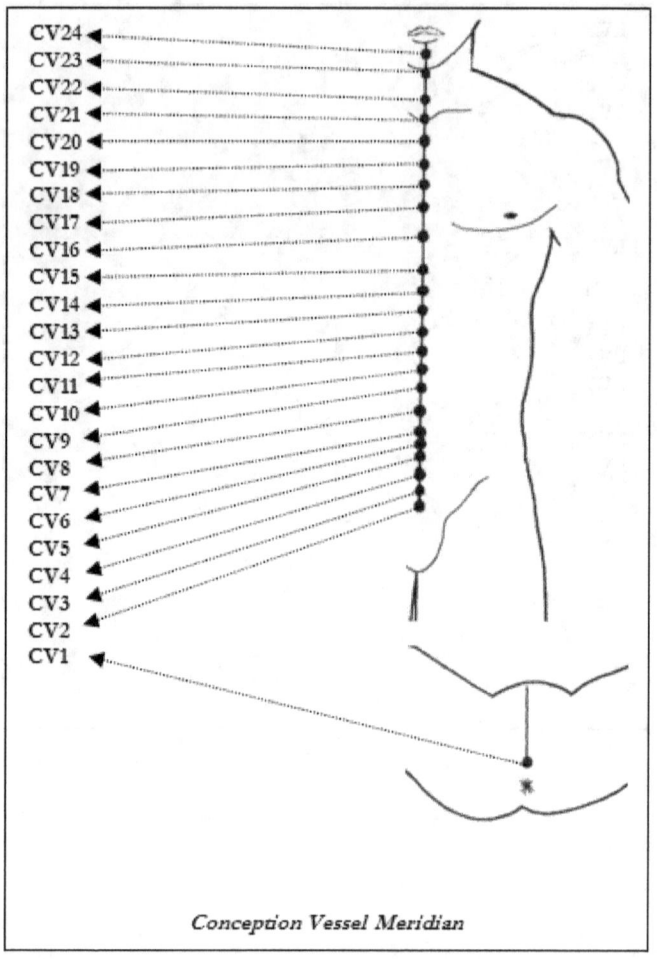

*Conception Vessel Meridian*

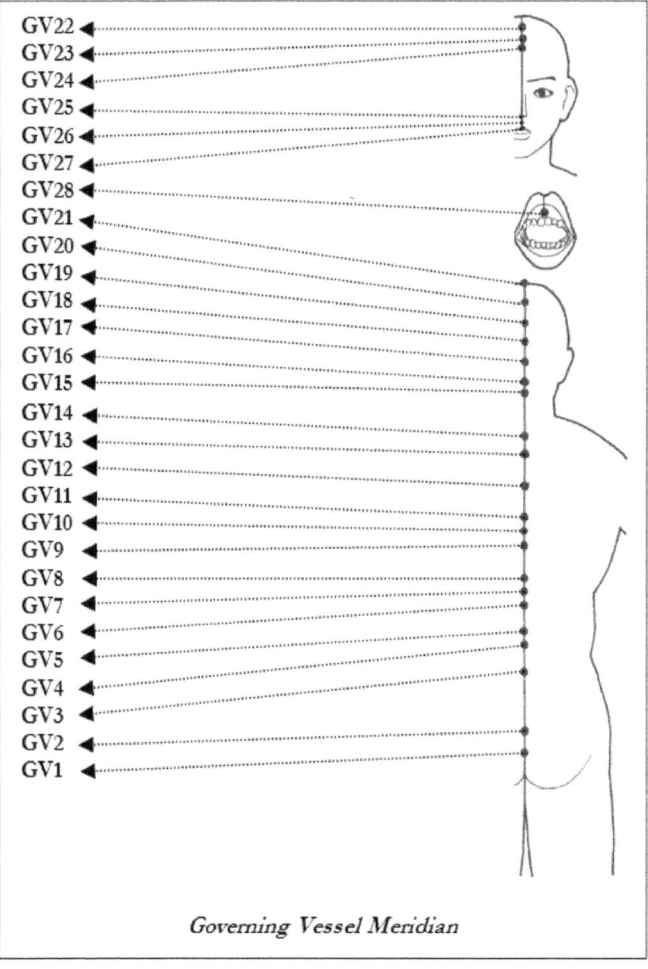

*Governing Vessel Meridian*

# ABOUT THE AUTHOR

Dr. Krishna N. Sharma born in Muhammadabad Gohana, District Mau, U.P., India on December 24th is an Author, Medical Professional and Educator. He is founder Editor of the Scientific Research Journal of India and founder Gen. Secretary of the Online Physio Community, India. He writes health articles and columns in various newspapers and magazines of India and Bangladesh. So far he has written and edited 39 books and has made 2 world records.

## AUTHOR CONTACT

Dr. L. Sharma Campus, Muhammadabad Gohana, Mau, U.P. 276403, India
Ph: +91-9320699167, 9305835734
Email: dr.krisharma@gmail.com
Web: http://www.krishna.info.ms

DR. KRISHNA N. SHARMA